MEDITERRANEAN MEALS MADE EASY FOR SENIORS

A Beginner's Guide:

Scientifically Backed Recipes to Reduce Cholesterol, Improve Brain Health, Lower Inflammation, Improve Digestion, Boost Longevity, One Delicious Meal at a Time

LifeQuest Publishing

INTRODUCTION

At LifeQuest Publishing, we understand that maintaining health and vitality becomes increasingly important as we age. Embracing the Mediterranean lifestyle offers a delightful and effective way to support your well-being.

Why Choose the Mediterranean Way?

The Mediterranean lifestyle emphasizes:

- Fresh Produce: Incorporating a variety of fruits and vegetables provides essential vitamins and antioxidants.
- Whole Grains: Foods like brown rice and whole-grain bread offer fiber and sustained energy.
- Healthy Fats: Using olive oil and enjoying nuts and seeds contributes to heart health
- Lean Proteins: Including fish and legumes supports muscle maintenance and overall health.

This approach not only nourishes the body but also encourages social interaction and mindful eating, enhancing overall quality of life.

Benefits for Seniors

Adopting the Mediterranean lifestyle can offer numerous advantages:

- Heart Health: Reducing the risk of cardiovascular diseases.
- Cognitive Support: Potentially lowering the risk of cognitive decline.
- Weight Management: Promoting a healthy weight through balanced eating.
- Bone Strength: Supporting bone density with nutrient-rich foods.
- Digestive Health: Enhancing digestion with high-fiber foods.

Getting Started

Transitioning to this lifestyle is simple and enjoyable:

- Plan Meals: Create weekly menus featuring Mediterranean-inspired dishes.
- Shop Smart: Focus on purchasing fresh, whole foods.
- Cook Together: Involve family or friends in meal preparation for added enjoyment.
- Stay Active: Incorporate regular physical activity to complement your diet.

Embracing the Mediterranean lifestyle is a joyful journey towards better health. At LifeQuest Publishing, we're here to support you every step of the way.

AUTHOR'S NOTE

At LifeQuest Publishing, our mission has always been to empower individuals to lead healthier, more fulfilling lives at every stage. As we age, the importance of nourishing our bodies and minds becomes even more paramount. This belief inspired us to create a guide tailored specifically for seniors, focusing on the Mediterranean lifestyle—a time-tested approach renowned for its health benefits and emphasis on fresh, wholesome foods.

In creating this book, our goal was to offer more than just dietary recommendations. We aimed to provide a comprehensive guide that celebrates not only nutritious eating but also the pleasures of cooking, the significance of community, and the joy found in savoring each moment. Our recipes are thoughtfully designed to be approachable for beginners, making the journey toward healthier eating both enjoyable and accessible for all.

We understand that transitioning to a new way of eating can be daunting. However, the Mediterranean approach is not about strict rules but about embracing balance, variety, and enjoyment in meals. It's about rediscovering the pleasure of food and the connections it fosters.

We hope this guide serves as a trusted companion on your journey to better health and well-being. May it inspire you to explore new flavors, share meals with loved ones, and embrace the vibrant life that the Mediterranean lifestyle offers.
With heartfelt thanks,
Your LifeQuest Publishing Family

Copyright © 2025 by LifeQuest Publishing
All rights reserved.
No part of this book may be reproduced in any form or by any electronic or mechanical means, including information storage and retrieval systems, without written permission from the author, except for the use of brief quotations in a book review.

TABLE OF CONTENTS

Introduction 2
Author's Note 5
What is the Mediterranean Diet? 6
A Rich History and Cultural Significance 6
Core Ingredients That Nourish 6
Health Benefits Backed by Science 7
Why It's Perfect for Seniors and Beginners 7
How to Use This Book 7

RECIPE SECTION
    GREEK YOGURT WITH HONEY AND WALNUTS 8
    MEDITERRANEAN VEGGIE OMELET 9
    AVOCADO TOAST WITH FETA AND TOMATOES 10
    OLIVE OIL BANANA BREAD 11
    BREAKFAST COUSCOUS WITH DRIED FRUITS 12
    TOMATO & SPINACH EGG MUFFINS 13
    WHOLE GRAIN PITA WITH HUMMUS AND CUCUMBERS 14
    SCRAMBLED EGGS WITH FRESH HERBS 15
    OVERNIGHT OATS WITH FIGS AND ALMONDS 16
    SMOOTHIE WITH BERRIES, YOGURT, AND CHIA SEEDS 17
    GREEK LEMON CHICKEN SOUP (AVGOLEMONO) 18
    HEARTY LENTIL AND SPINACH SOUP 19
    TOMATO BASIL CHICKPEA STEW 20
    MEDITERRANEAN FISH STEW 21
    WHITE BEAN AND KALE SOUP 22
    EGGPLANT AND ZUCCHINI STEW 23
    SPICED CARROT AND RED LENTIL SOUP 24
    LEMON GARLIC CHICKEN STEW 25
    SLOW-COOKED MOROCCAN LAMB STEW 26
    CAULIFLOWER AND CHICKPEA SOUP 27
    CLASSIC GREEK SALAD 28
    QUINOA AND ROASTED VEGETABLE SALAD 29
    CUCUMBER, TOMATO, AND RED ONION SALAD 30
    CHICKPEA AND TUNA SALAD 31
    LENTIL SALAD WITH FETA AND HERBS 32
    ARUGULA SALAD WITH PEARS AND WALNUTS 33
    CAPRESE SALAD WITH BALSAMIC GLAZE 34
    MEDITERRANEAN ORZO SALAD 35
    BEET AND FETA SALAD 36

COUSCOUS SALAD WITH LEMON AND MINT	37
STUFFED BELL PEPPERS WITH RICE AND HERBS	38
EGGPLANT PARMESAN (BAKED, NOT FRIED)	39
GRILLED HALLOUMI WITH VEGETABLES	40
RATATOUILLE WITH OLIVE OIL AND BASIL	41
SPINACH AND FETA STUFFED PORTOBELLOS	42
CHICKPEA AND SWEET POTATO CURRY	43
MUSHROOM AND ZUCCHINI STIR-FRY	44
FALAFEL WITH YOGURT SAUCE	45
BAKED FETA WITH CHERRY TOMATOES	46
LENTIL AND VEGGIE PATTIES	47
GRILLED LEMON HERB SALMON	48
BAKED COD WITH TOMATOES AND OLIVES	49
SHRIMP SKEWERS WITH GARLIC AND PAPRIKA	50
MEDITERRANEAN TUNA PATTIES	51
SARDINES WITH LEMON AND PARSLEY	52
FISH TACOS WITH YOGURT DILL SAUCE	53
MUSSELS IN TOMATO WINE BROTH	54
GREEK-STYLE GRILLED OCTOPUS	55
SEARED MAHI MAHI WITH MANGO SALSA	56
BAKED TROUT WITH HERBS AND LEMON	57
GARLIC BUTTER SHRIMP AND ZOODLES	58
PAN-SEARED SCALLOPS WITH SPINACH	59
SALMON WITH CUCUMBER-DILL SAUCE	60
TUNA AND WHITE BEAN SKILLET	61
ANCHOVY AND ROASTED PEPPER FLATBREAD	62
LEMON OREGANO GRILLED CHICKEN	63
BAKED CHICKEN WITH TOMATOES AND CAPERS	64
GROUND TURKEY AND VEGGIE SKILLET	65
CHICKEN WITH ARTICHOKES AND OLIVES	66
RECIPE NAME: HERBED CHICKEN THIGHS WITH COUSCOUS	67
TURKEY AND QUINOA STUFFED ZUCCHINI	68
CHICKEN SHAWARMA BOWLS	69
GREEK MEATBALLS (KEFTEDES)	70
GRILLED CHICKEN WITH TZATZIKI	71
CHICKEN AND SPINACH STUFFED PEPPERS	72
ROSEMARY GARLIC TURKEY CUTLETS	73
MEDITERRANEAN CHICKEN AND LENTILS	74
CHICKEN AND EGGPLANT BAKE	75

SPICY CHICKEN WITH ROASTED VEGETABLES	76
WHOLE WHEAT SPAGHETTI WITH CHERRY TOMATOES & BASIL	77
ORZO WITH ROASTED PEPPERS AND SPINACH	78
CHICKPEA AND OLIVE PASTA	79
BROWN RICE WITH GRILLED VEGETABLES	80
LENTIL AND TOMATO RICE BOWL	81
BARLEY RISOTTO WITH MUSHROOMS	82
COUSCOUS WITH CHICKPEAS AND CARROTS	83
QUINOA AND LEMON PILAF	84
BULGUR WHEAT WITH HERBS AND FETA	85
FARRO SALAD WITH TOMATOES AND OLIVES	86
CLASSIC HUMMUS WITH OLIVE OIL	87
TZATZIKI CUCUMBER YOGURT DIP	88
ROASTED EGGPLANT DIP (BABA GANOUSH)	89
GRILLED ZUCCHINI WITH MINT	90
SPICED ROASTED CHICKPEAS	91
MARINATED OLIVES WITH LEMON AND GARLIC	92
GARLIC ROASTED CAULIFLOWER	93
MEDITERRANEAN ROASTED POTATOES	94
BAKED FETA AND OLIVES	95
PITA CHIPS WITH ZA'ATAR	96
STUFFED GRAPE LEAVES (DOLMAS)	97
MINI GREEK VEGGIE WRAPS	98
ROASTED RED PEPPER AND GOAT CHEESE TOASTS	99
HERB AND OLIVE TAPENADE	100
SPICED ALMONDS WITH SEA SALT	101
YOGURT WITH HONEY, FIGS, AND PISTACHIOS	102
ALMOND OLIVE OIL CAKE	103
BAKED PEARS WITH WALNUTS AND CINNAMON	104
SEMOLINA ORANGE CAKE (LOW-SUGAR)	105
FRESH FRUIT SALAD WITH MINT AND LEMON	106
30-Day Mediterranean Meal Plan	107
Week One	108
Week Two	109
Week Three	110
Week Four	111
Conclusion	112

WHAT IS THE MEDITERRANEAN DIET?

The Mediterranean diet isn't a fad or a rigid eating plan – it's a way of life. Rooted in the traditional eating habits of countries bordering the Mediterranean Sea, this diet emphasizes fresh, seasonal, and whole foods enjoyed in balance. From Greece to Italy, Spain to southern France, the Mediterranean lifestyle focuses on simplicity, flavor, and nourishing the body through real food.

At its heart, the Mediterranean diet is about enjoying meals with loved ones, eating more plants and fewer processed foods, and making every bite both delicious and beneficial for your health.

A RICH HISTORY AND CULTURAL SIGNIFICANCE

The Mediterranean diet is inspired by centuries-old culinary traditions from coastal regions where people historically lived longer and healthier lives. Meals weren't just about feeding the body – they were social rituals filled with family, laughter, and love. Bread was dipped in olive oil, fresh vegetables were harvested from backyard gardens, and fish was often caught the same day it was served.

This time-honored approach to food has drawn attention from nutritionists and medical experts alike. In fact, UNESCO has recognized the Mediterranean diet as an Intangible Cultural Heritage of Humanity, highlighting its powerful blend of nutrition, culture, and lifestyle.

CORE INGREDIENTS THAT NOURISH

The Mediterranean diet focuses on wholesome ingredients that are easy to find and prepare. These core components form the foundation of every recipe in this book:

- Olive oil – rich in heart-healthy fats
- Whole grains – brown rice, quinoa, farro, whole wheat pasta
- Legumes – chickpeas, lentils, beans
- Fruits & vegetables – fresh, seasonal, and colorful
- Lean proteins – fish, chicken, turkey, eggs
- Nuts & seeds – almonds, walnuts, flaxseeds
- Herbs & spices – basil, oregano, garlic, parsley, mint
- Dairy in moderation – Greek yogurt, cheese like feta and parmesan

There's no need for complicated ingredients – just real, honest food prepared with care.

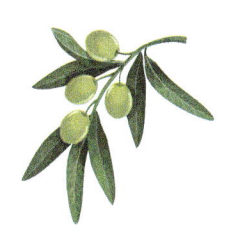

HEALTH BENEFITS BACKED BY SCIENCE

The Mediterranean diet is one of the most studied and recommended eating patterns by healthcare professionals. Its benefits are impressive and well-documented:

- Supports heart health by lowering LDL ("bad") cholesterol
- Helps reduce inflammation throughout the body
- Promotes healthy brain aging and lowers risk of cognitive decline
- Contributes to weight management and improved digestion
- Lowers the risk of chronic illnesses like diabetes and certain cancers
- Encourages longer lifespan and better overall well-being

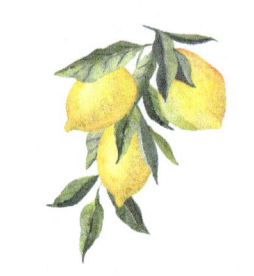

WHY IT'S PERFECT FOR SENIORS AND BEGINNERS

This book was designed with simplicity in mind. Whether you're new to cooking or just looking for recipes that don't require complicated steps, you'll find each dish approachable, nutritious, and full of flavor. For seniors, the Mediterranean diet is gentle on digestion, supportive of heart and brain health, and encourages foods that are easy to prepare and enjoy without heavy sauces or hard-to-chew textures.

Plus, the focus on anti-inflammatory ingredients can help with joint health, energy levels, and vitality at any age.

HOW TO USE THIS BOOK

& Kitchen Essentials for Mediterranean Cooking

This cookbook features 100 carefully selected recipes and a complete meal plan to guide you through weeks of healthy, satisfying meals. Each section is divided into breakfasts, soups, mains, snacks, and more, with clear instructions and wholesome ingredients you can find at any local grocery store.

To get the most out of your Mediterranean kitchen, stock these essentials:

- Extra-virgin olive oil
- Lemons and garlic
- Whole grains like quinoa, bulgur, and brown rice
- Canned beans and tomatoes
- Greek yogurt and feta cheese
- Dried herbs and spices (oregano, thyme, cinnamon, cumin)
- Fresh vegetables like spinach, tomatoes, and bell peppers
- Frozen fish or seafood for convenience
- Whole wheat pasta or couscous

This book is your guide to living well – one tasty, nourishing meal at a time.

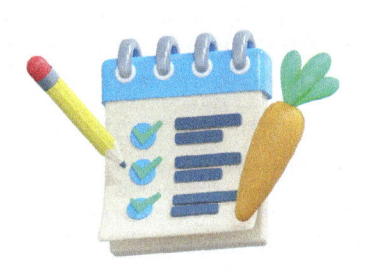

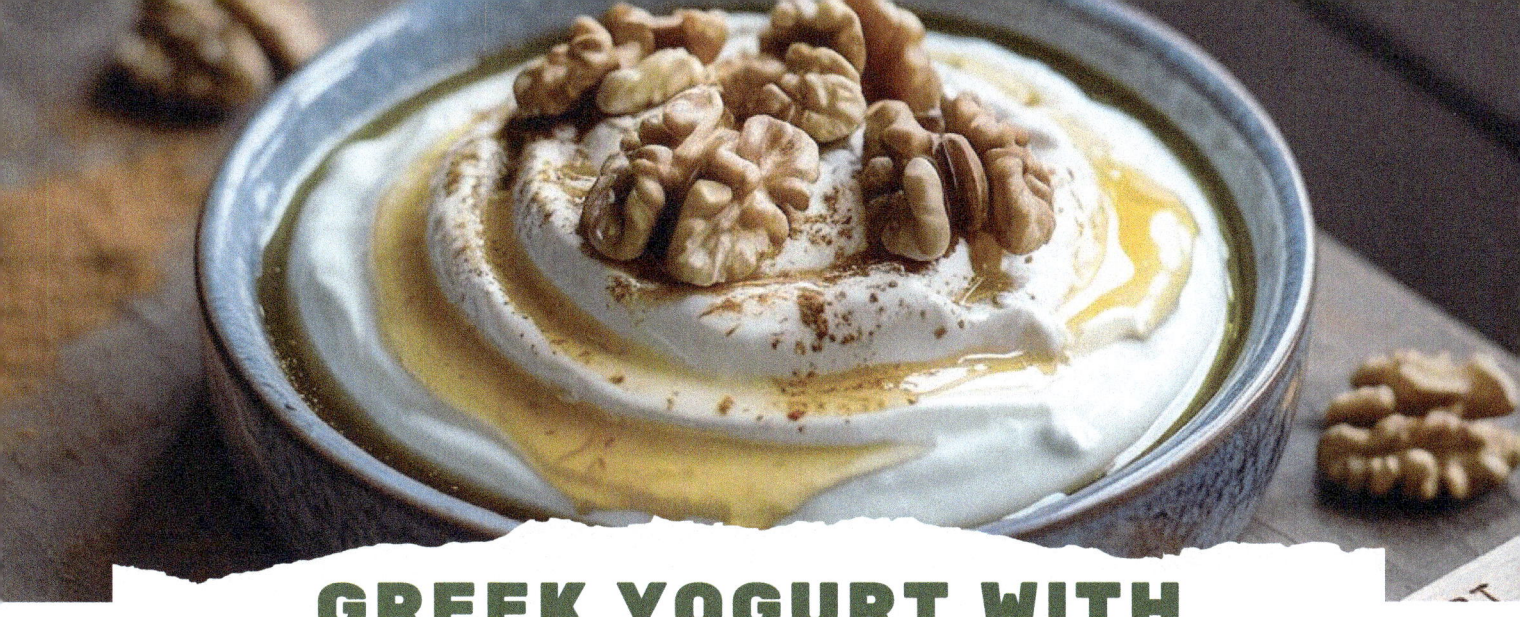

GREEK YOGURT WITH HONEY AND WALNUTS

Servings: 2   **Total Time:** 5 Min

Calories: 210 | **Protein:** 10g | **Fat:** 10g | **Carbohydrates:** 20g

Ingredients

- 1 cup plain Greek yogurt (full-fat or low-fat)
- 2 tablespoons honey
- ¼ cup walnut halves, roughly chopped
- 1 pinch ground cinnamon (optional)

Directions

- Mix awesome and fun together.
- Add a dash of color.
- Flavor everything, divide the Greek yogurt evenly into two serving bowls.
- Drizzle 1 tablespoon of honey over each bowl of yogurt.
- Sprinkle chopped walnuts on top.
- (Optional) Add a light dusting of ground cinnamon for extra warmth and flavor.
- Serve immediately and enjoy!

Tips

- For extra crunch, lightly toast the walnuts before adding.
- You can substitute maple syrup for honey if desired.
- Add fresh berries for a fruit-filled twist.
- This recipe makes a great healthy dessert or energizing breakfast.

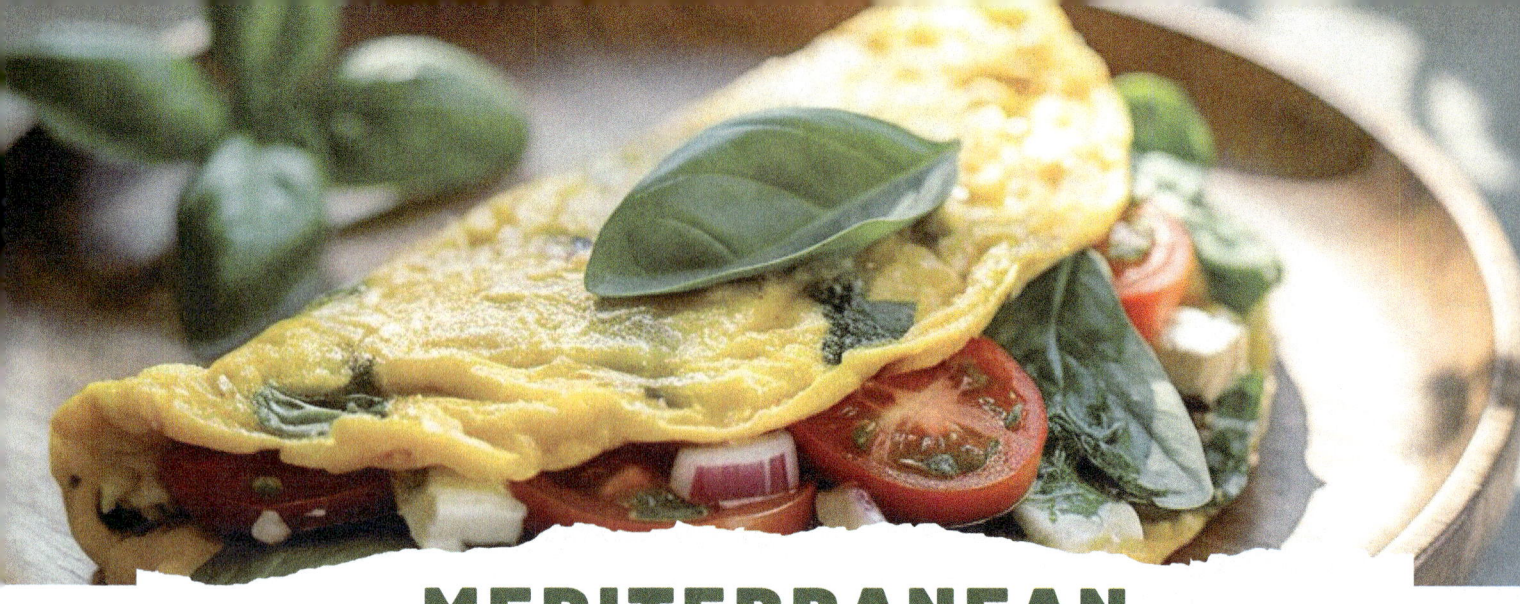

MEDITERRANEAN VEGGIE OMELET

Servings: 1 | **Total Time:** 15 Min

Calories: 250 | **Protein:** 14g | **Carbohydrates:** 6g | **Fat:** 18g

Ingredients

- 2 large eggs
- 2 tablespoons milk (optional, for fluffiness)
- 1 tablespoon olive oil
- ¼ cup diced tomatoes
- ¼ cup chopped baby spinach
- 2 tablespoons chopped red onion
- 2 tablespoons crumbled feta cheese
- Salt and black pepper to taste
- A pinch of dried oregano (optional)

Directions

- In a small bowl, whisk together the eggs, milk, salt, pepper, and oregano until well combined.
- Heat olive oil in a non-stick skillet over medium heat.
- Sauté the onions for 1–2 minutes until they begin to soften.
- Add spinach and tomatoes; cook for another 1–2 minutes until the spinach wilts slightly.
- Pour the egg mixture over the vegetables, tilting the pan to spread it evenly.
- Cook for 3–4 minutes or until the edges set. Sprinkle feta cheese on top.
- Carefully fold the omelet in half and cook for another minute until fully cooked through.
- Slide onto a plate and serve warm.

Tips

- For extra flavor, add a few sliced olives or roasted red peppers.
- Use egg whites or a plant-based egg substitute if preferred.
- Serve with a side of whole-grain toast or fresh fruit for a complete breakfast.
- Make it a meal for two by doubling the ingredients.

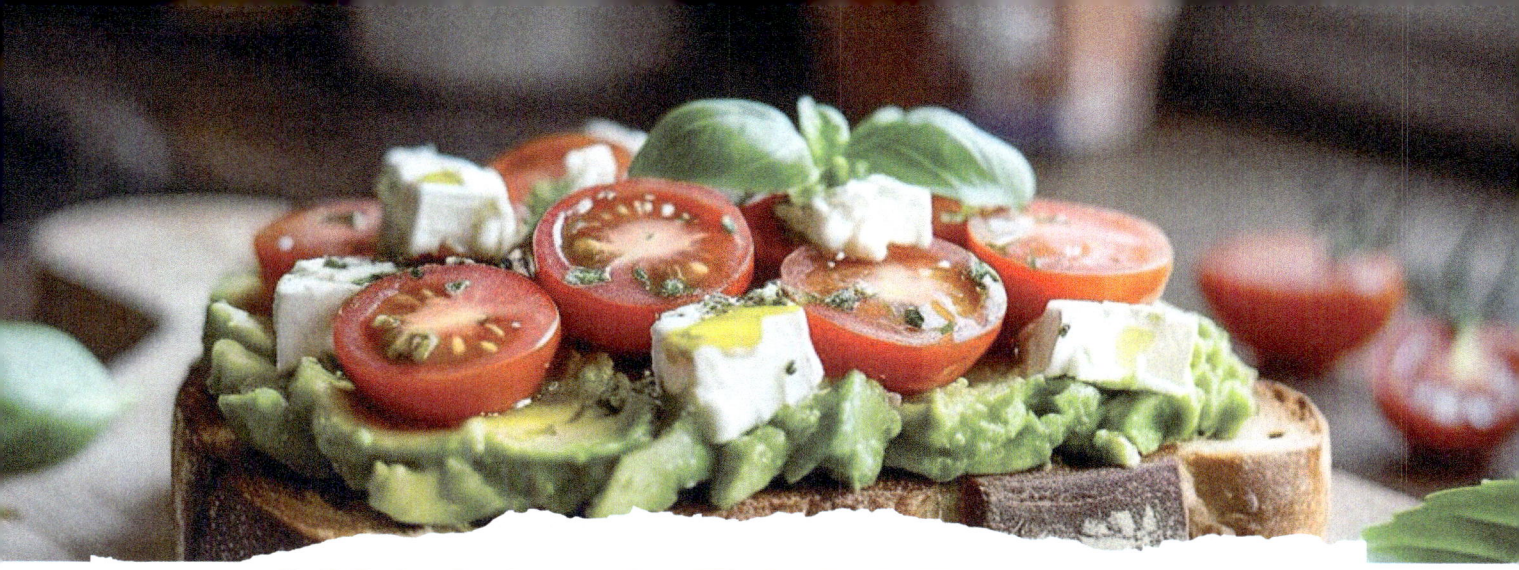

AVOCADO TOAST WITH FETA AND TOMATOES

Servings: 2   **Total Time:** 10 Min

Calories: 280 | **Protein:** 7g | **Carbohydrates:** 22g | **Fat:** 20g

Ingredients

- 2 slices whole grain or sourdough bread
- 1 ripe avocado
- ½ cup cherry tomatoes, halved
- ¼ cup crumbled feta cheese
- 1 tbsp extra-virgin olive oil
- ½ tsp lemon juice
- Salt and black pepper, to taste
- Optional: chopped fresh basil or parsley for garnish

Directions

- Toast the bread slices to your desired crispness.
- Cut the avocado in half, remove the pit, and scoop the flesh into a small bowl.
- Mash the avocado with a fork and mix in lemon juice, a pinch of salt, and black pepper.
- Spread the mashed avocado evenly over each toast slice.
- Top with halved cherry tomatoes and sprinkle with crumbled feta cheese.
- Drizzle a little olive oil over each slice and garnish with fresh herbs if using.
- Serve immediately.

Tips

- Use multi-seed or sprouted bread for added texture and nutrients.
- Add a pinch of red pepper flakes for a spicy kick.
- For extra protein, top with a poached or boiled egg.
- This makes a great light lunch or a filling breakfast.

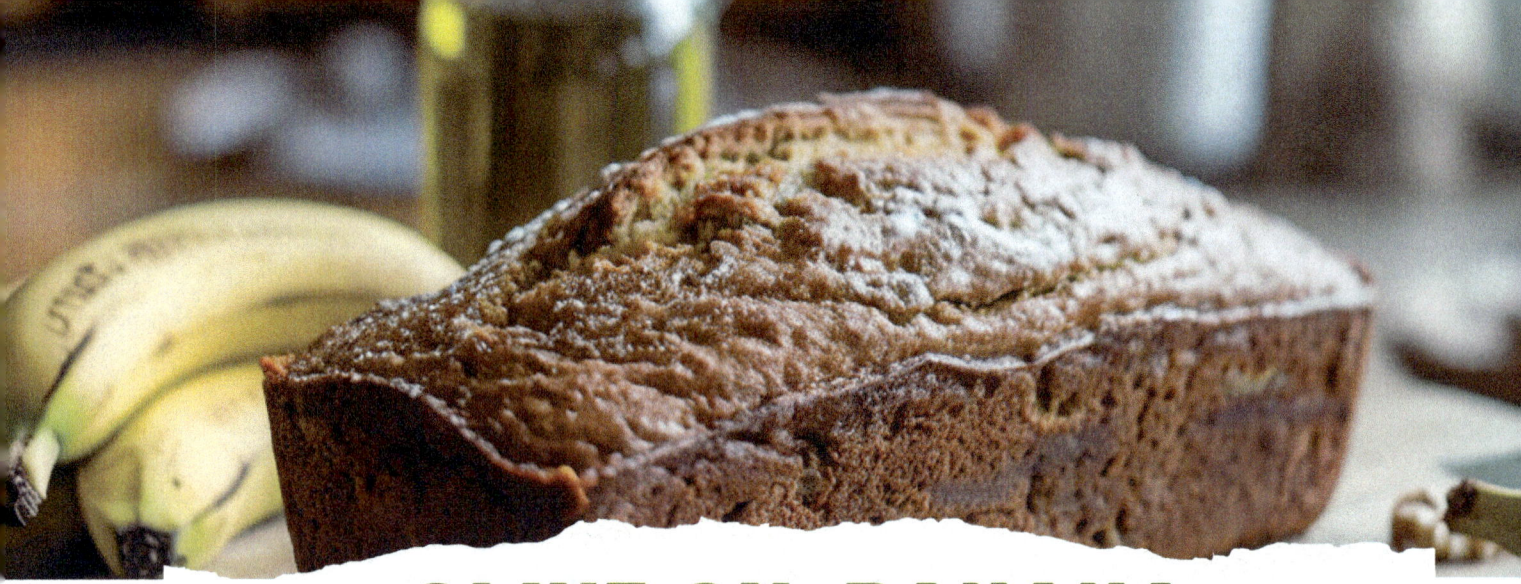

OLIVE OIL BANANA BREAD

Servings: 8   **Total Time:** 55 Min

Calories: 190 | **Protein:** 4g | **Carbohydrates:** 28g | **Sugars:** 12g

Ingredients

- 3 ripe bananas, mashed
- 2 large eggs
- 1/3 cup extra-virgin olive oil
- 1/2 cup honey or maple syrup
- 1/4 cup plain Greek yogurt
- 1 tsp vanilla extract
- 1 1/2 cups whole wheat flour
- 1 tsp baking soda
- 1/2 tsp salt
- 1/2 tsp cinnamon (optional)
- 1/4 cup chopped walnuts (optional)

Tips

- For extra moisture, use very ripe bananas with brown spots.
- Add a handful of dark chocolate chips for a sweeter twist.
- This bread freezes well. Slice and wrap individually for quick snacks.
- You can substitute whole wheat flour with a 50/50 mix of all-purpose and whole wheat for a lighter texture.

Directions

- Preheat your oven to 350°F (175°C). Lightly grease a 9x5-inch loaf pan or line with parchment paper.
- In a large mixing bowl, combine mashed bananas, eggs, olive oil, honey (or maple syrup), Greek yogurt, and vanilla extract. Stir until smooth.
- In another bowl, mix the flour, baking soda, salt, and cinnamon (if using).
- Gradually add the dry ingredients to the wet mixture. Stir gently until just combined. Do not overmix.
- Fold in chopped walnuts if using.
- Pour the batter into the prepared loaf pan and smooth the top.
- Bake for 45–50 minutes, or until a toothpick inserted into the center comes out clean.
- Let cool in the pan for 10 minutes, then transfer to a wire rack to cool completely before slicing.

BREAKFAST COUSCOUS WITH DRIED FRUITS

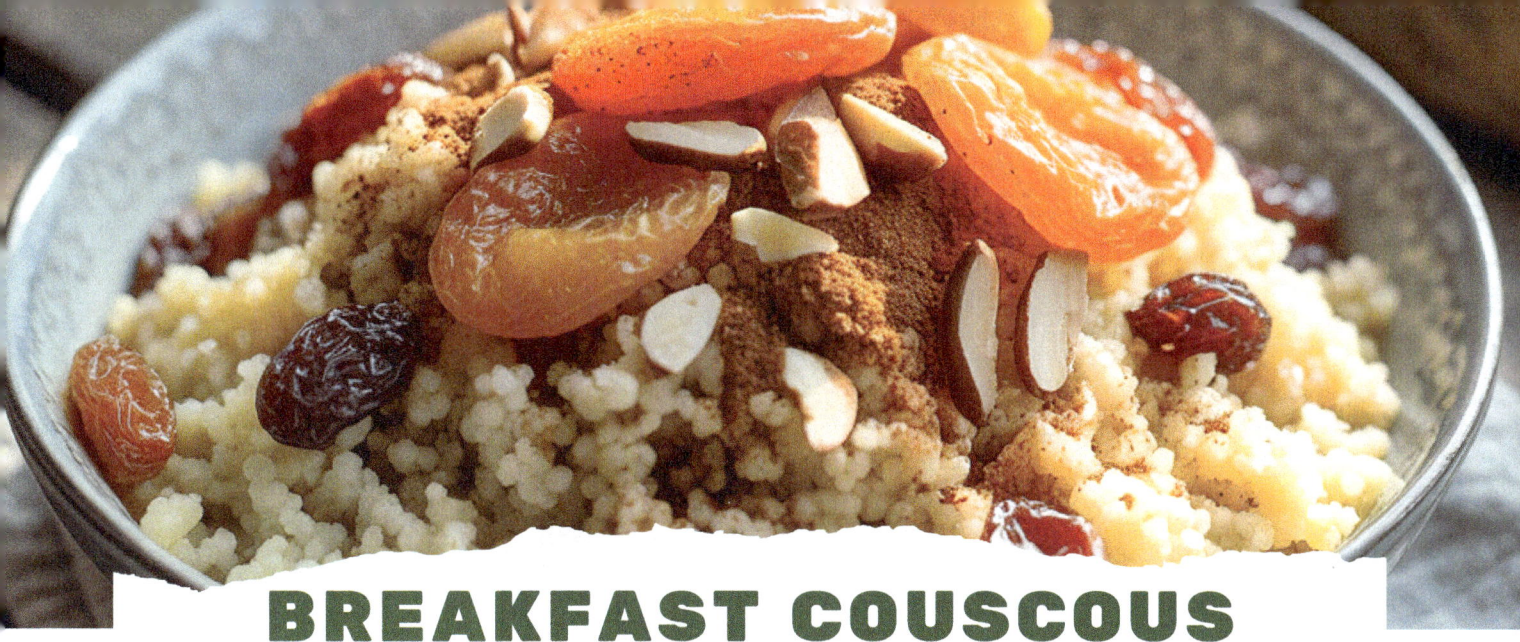

Servings: 2 | **Total Time:** 15 Min

Calories: ~280 | **Protein:** 6g | **Carbohydrates:** 50g **Sugars:** 14g | **Fat:** 6g

Ingredients

- 1 cup whole wheat couscous
- 1 cup water
- ¼ cup chopped dried apricots
- 2 tablespoons raisins or chopped dates
- 1 tablespoon honey or maple syrup
- ½ teaspoon ground cinnamon
- ½ cup low-fat milk or plant-based milk (optional)
- 1 tablespoon chopped almonds or walnuts (optional)
- Pinch of salt

Directions

- In a small pot, bring the water and a pinch of salt to a boil.
- Stir in the couscous, dried apricots, and raisins. Remove from heat and cover. Let sit for 5 minutes.
- Fluff the couscous with a fork, then stir in the honey (or maple syrup) and cinnamon.
- Divide into two bowls and drizzle with milk if desired. Top with chopped nuts for added crunch.
- Serve warm and enjoy!

Tips

- For extra flavor, try cooking the couscous in low-fat milk instead of water.
- Swap in your favorite dried fruits, like figs or cranberries.
- Add a dollop of Greek yogurt on top for added creaminess and protein.

TOMATO & SPINACH EGG MUFFINS

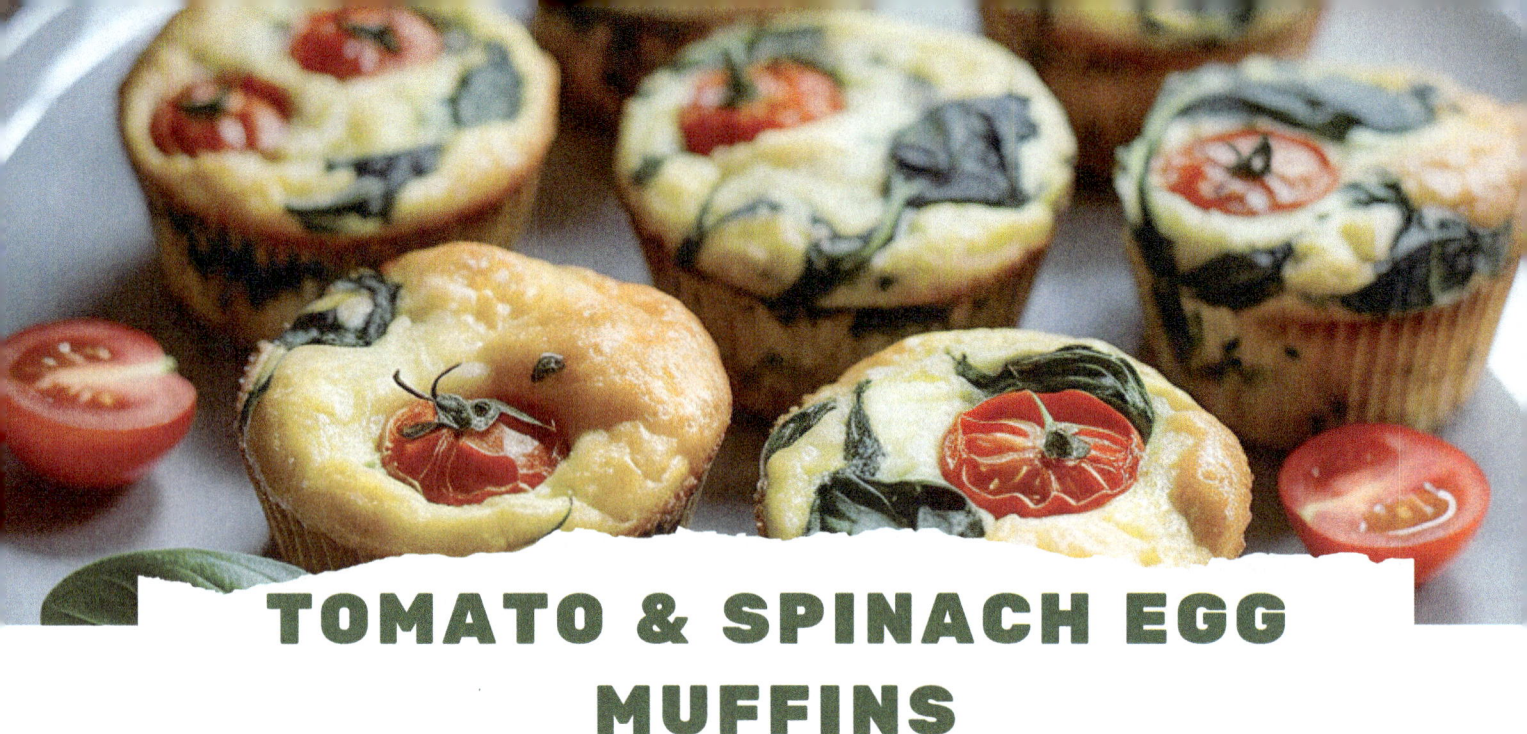

Servings: 6   **Total Time:** 25 Min

Calories: 140 | **Protein:** 11g | **Fat:** 9g | **Carbohydrates:** 2g

Ingredients

- 6 large eggs
- 1/4 cup milk (or unsweetened almond milk)
- 1 cup fresh spinach, chopped
- 1/2 cup cherry tomatoes, halved
- 1/4 cup feta cheese, crumbled (optional)
- 1/4 tsp salt
- 1/4 tsp black pepper
- 1/2 tsp dried oregano (optional)
- Olive oil or cooking spray (for greasing the muffin tin)

Directions

- Preheat your oven to 375°F (190°C). Lightly grease a 6-cup muffin tin with olive oil or cooking spray.
- In a medium bowl, whisk together the eggs and milk until well combined.
- Add chopped spinach, cherry tomatoes, salt, pepper, and oregano to the egg mixture. Stir well.
- Pour the mixture evenly into the muffin cups. Top each with a sprinkle of feta cheese, if using.
- Bake for 18–20 minutes, or until the egg muffins are set and lightly golden on top.
- Let cool for 5 minutes before removing from the tin. Serve warm or store in the fridge for up to 4 days.

Tips

- These are perfect for meal prep – just reheat in the microwave for a quick breakfast or snack.
- Swap in other veggies like bell peppers or mushrooms based on what you have on hand.
- For added flavor, sprinkle with fresh herbs like parsley or basil before serving.

WHOLE GRAIN PITA WITH HUMMUS AND CUCUMBERS

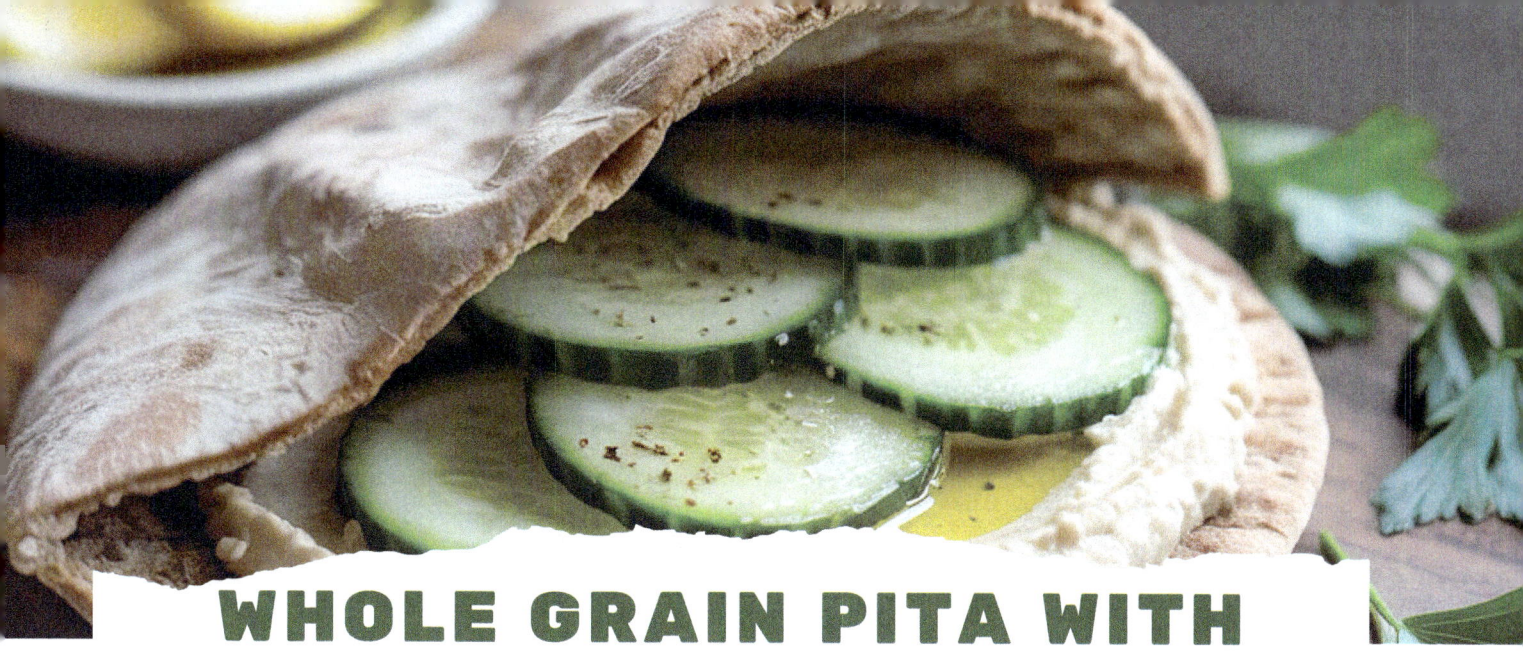

Servings: 2 **Total Time:** 10 Min

Calories: 230 | **Protein:** 7g | **Carbohydrates:** 28g | **Sodium:** 240mg

Ingredients

- 2 whole grain pita pockets
- ½ cup hummus (store-bought or homemade)
- 1 cup cucumber, thinly sliced
- ¼ teaspoon ground black pepper
- 1 tablespoon extra-virgin olive oil (optional)
- 1 teaspoon lemon juice
- Fresh parsley or mint leaves for garnish (optional)

Directions

- Slice each pita pocket in half and gently open the pockets.
- Spread 2 tablespoons of hummus inside each half.
- Layer cucumber slices evenly inside the pita over the hummus.
- Drizzle a few drops of olive oil and lemon juice inside each pocket for added flavor.
- Sprinkle with ground black pepper.
- Garnish with chopped parsley or mint if desired.
- Serve immediately and enjoy!

Tips

- Swap cucumbers for thinly sliced bell peppers or tomatoes for variety.
- Use flavored hummus (like roasted red pepper or garlic) to change up the flavor.
- Lightly warm the pita in a toaster for a softer texture.
- Ideal as a light lunch, snack, or part of a Mediterranean mezze platter.

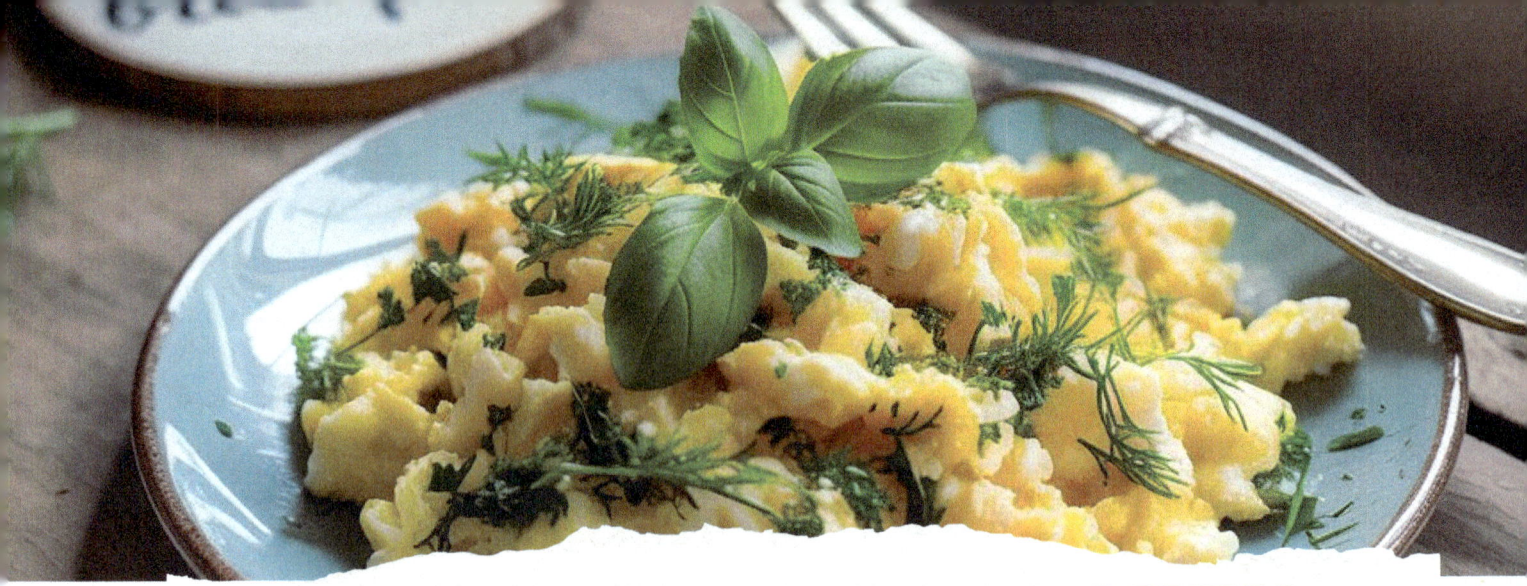

SCRAMBLED EGGS WITH FRESH HERBS

Servings: 2 **Total Time:** 10 Min

Calories: 170 | **Protein:** 11g | **Carbohydrates:** 2g | **Fat:** 13g

Ingredients

- 4 large eggs
- 2 tablespoons milk (optional, for creamier texture)
- 1 tablespoon olive oil or unsalted butter
- 2 tablespoons chopped fresh herbs (such as parsley, chives, dill, or basil)
- Salt and pepper to taste

Directions

- Crack the eggs into a bowl, add milk (if using), and beat well with a fork or whisk until fully combined.
- Stir in the chopped fresh herbs, reserving a pinch for garnish.
- Heat olive oil or butter in a non-stick skillet over medium-low heat.
- Pour in the egg mixture and let it sit undisturbed for a few seconds.
- ·Gently stir with a spatula, scraping the eggs from the edges toward the center as they begin to set.
- Cook until softly scrambled and slightly creamy, then remove from heat.
- Season with salt and pepper. Garnish with remaining herbs and serve warm.

Tips

- For fluffier eggs, beat in a bit of air while whisking.
- Use a mix of herbs for a brighter flavor – parsley for freshness, chives for a light onion taste, and dill for a hint of sweetness.
- Cook on low heat for soft, creamy eggs; high heat can make them rubbery.
- Great served with whole grain toast or sliced avocado on the side.

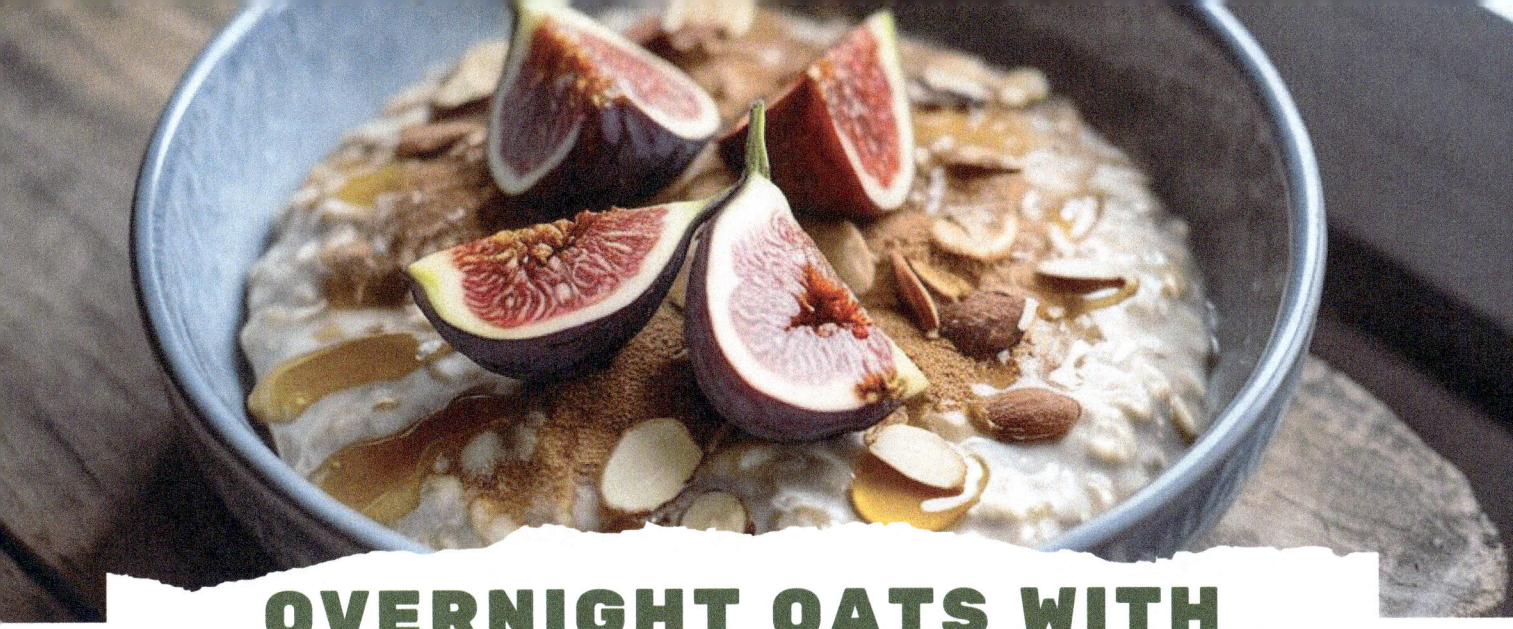

OVERNIGHT OATS WITH FIGS AND ALMONDS

Servings: 2   **Total Time:** 10 Min

Calories: 280 | **Protein:** 10g | **Carbohydrates:** 35g | **Fat:** 10g

Ingredients

- 1 cup rolled oats
- 1 cup unsweetened almond milk (or any milk of choice)
- ½ cup plain Greek yogurt
- 2 dried figs, chopped (or fresh if available)
- 2 tablespoons chopped almonds
- 1 tablespoon honey or maple syrup (optional)
- ½ teaspoon ground cinnamon
- Pinch of salt

Directions

- In a medium bowl or mason jar, combine oats, almond milk, Greek yogurt, cinnamon, and salt. Stir well.
- Add the chopped figs and almonds, mixing them gently into the oat mixture.
- Drizzle in the honey or maple syrup if using, and stir to combine.
- Cover and refrigerate overnight (or for at least 4–6 hours).
- In the morning, give the oats a good stir and top with extra figs or almonds if desired. Enjoy chilled.

Tips

- Use fresh figs when in season for an extra juicy texture.
- For added creaminess, swap almond milk with oat milk or coconut milk.
- Want more protein? Add a tablespoon of chia seeds or a scoop of protein powder.
- These oats stay fresh for up to 3 days in the fridge – perfect for meal prep.

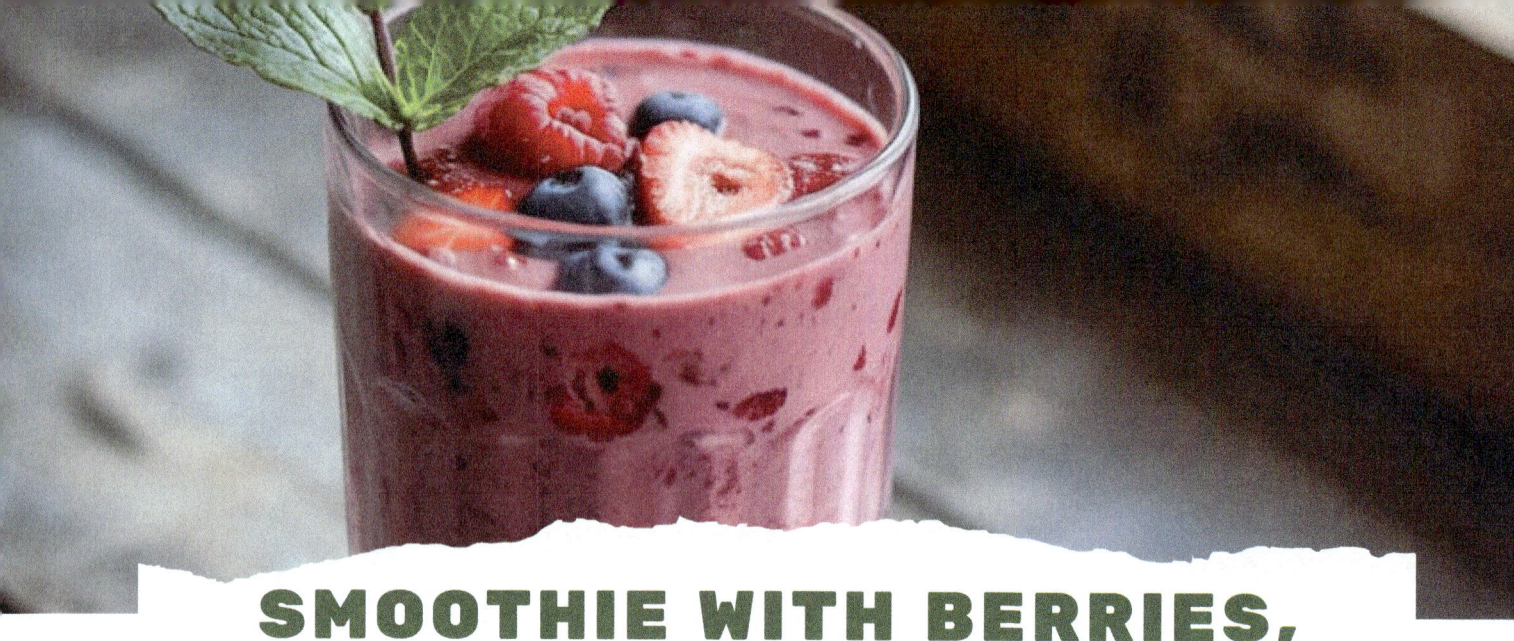

SMOOTHIE WITH BERRIES, YOGURT, AND CHIA SEEDS

Servings: 2   **Total Time:** 5 Min

Calories: 170 | **Protein:** 10g | **Fat:** 5g | **Carbohydrates:** 20g

Ingredients

- 1 cup mixed berries (fresh or frozen: strawberries, blueberries, raspberries)
- 1 cup plain Greek yogurt
- 1 tablespoon chia seeds
- 1 small banana (optional, for natural sweetness)
- ½ cup unsweetened almond milk (or milk of choice)
- 1 teaspoon honey or maple syrup (optional)
- ¼ teaspoon vanilla extract (optional)

Directions

- Add the berries, Greek yogurt, chia seeds, banana, and almond milk into a blender.
- Blend on high until smooth and creamy.
- Taste and adjust sweetness by adding honey or maple syrup if desired.
- Pour into two glasses and serve immediately.
- Garnish with a few extra berries or a sprinkle of chia seeds if you like.

Tips

- Use frozen berries for a thicker, frostier smoothie.
- Let the smoothie sit for 5–10 minutes to allow chia seeds to expand and thicken it naturally.
- Add a handful of spinach for extra nutrients – you won't even taste it!
- Make it dairy-free by swapping yogurt with coconut yogurt and using plant-based milk.

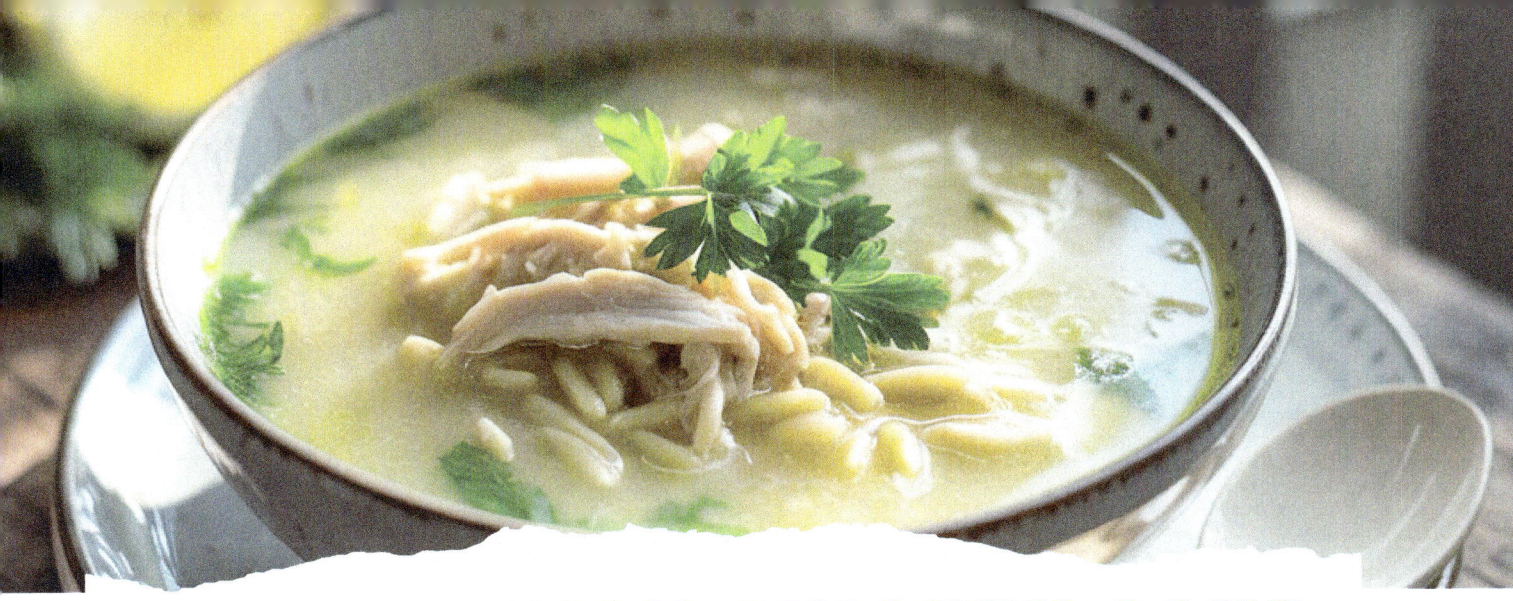

GREEK LEMON CHICKEN SOUP (AVGOLEMONO)

Servings: 4   **Total Time:** 35 Min

Calories: 280 | **Protein:** 24g | **Fat:** 10g | **Carbohydrates:** 20g

Ingredients

- 6 cups chicken broth
- 2 cups cooked, shredded chicken (preferably from bone-in breasts or thighs)
- ½ cup uncooked orzo or rice
- 3 large eggs
- ¼ cup fresh lemon juice (about 2 lemons)
- Salt and black pepper to taste
- 1 tablespoon chopped fresh dill or parsley (optional)

Directions

- In a large pot, bring the chicken broth to a boil. Add the orzo (or rice), reduce heat, and simmer until tender (about 10–12 minutes).
- Stir in the shredded chicken and simmer on low for another 3–5 minutes
- In a separate bowl, whisk the eggs until frothy. Slowly add the lemon juice while whisking to combine.
- Slowly ladle 1 cup of the hot broth (a little at a time) into the egg-lemon mixture, whisking constantly. This prevents the eggs from scrambling.
- Add Mixture to Soup: Turn off the heat and slowly stir the egg-lemon mixture into the soup. The broth will turn creamy without any cream.
- Season & Serve: Taste and season with salt and pepper.

Tips

- Don't boil the soup after adding the eggs—this keeps it smooth and silky.
- Use rotisserie chicken or leftover roast chicken to save time.
- Add extra lemon juice if you prefer a more tangy flavor.
- Make it gluten-free by using rice instead of orzo.
- This soup stores well and tastes even better the next day. Reheat gently to avoid curdling.

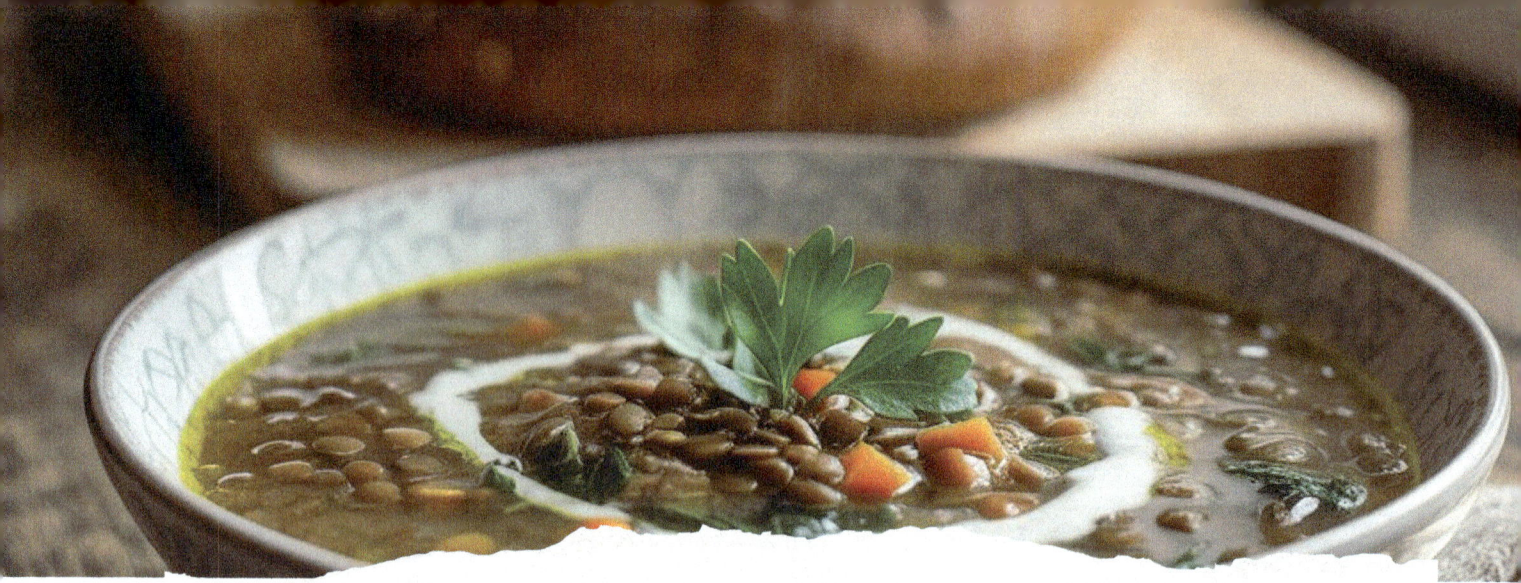

HEARTY LENTIL AND SPINACH SOUP

Servings: 4   **Total Time:** 40 Min

Calories: 230 | **Protein:** 14g | **Fat:** 4g | **Carbohydrates:** 36g

Ingredients

- 1 tablespoon extra-virgin olive oil
- 1 small onion, finely chopped
- 2 cloves garlic, minced
- 2 medium carrots, diced
- 2 celery stalks, diced
- 1 teaspoon ground cumin
- 1 cup dried brown or green lentils, rinsed
- 6 cups low-sodium vegetable broth or water
- 1 bay leaf
- Salt and black pepper to taste
- 4 cups fresh spinach (or 1 cup frozen spinach, thawed)
- Juice of ½ lemon

Directions

- Heat olive oil in a large pot over medium heat. Add the chopped onion, garlic, carrots, and celery. Sauté for 5–7 minutes, until softened.
- Stir in the cumin and cook for 1 more minute to release its flavor.
- Add the lentils, broth, and bay leaf. Bring to a boil, then reduce heat and simmer uncovered for 25–30 minutes, or until lentils are tender.
- Remove the bay leaf. Stir in the spinach and cook for another 2–3 minutes, just until wilted.
- Season with salt, black pepper, and a squeeze of lemon juice.
- Serve hot with a slice of whole grain bread, if desired.

Tips

- You can use red lentils for a quicker-cooking, softer texture.
- Add diced tomatoes or a pinch of red pepper flakes for extra flavor.
- This soup stores well and tastes even better the next day – perfect for meal prep!

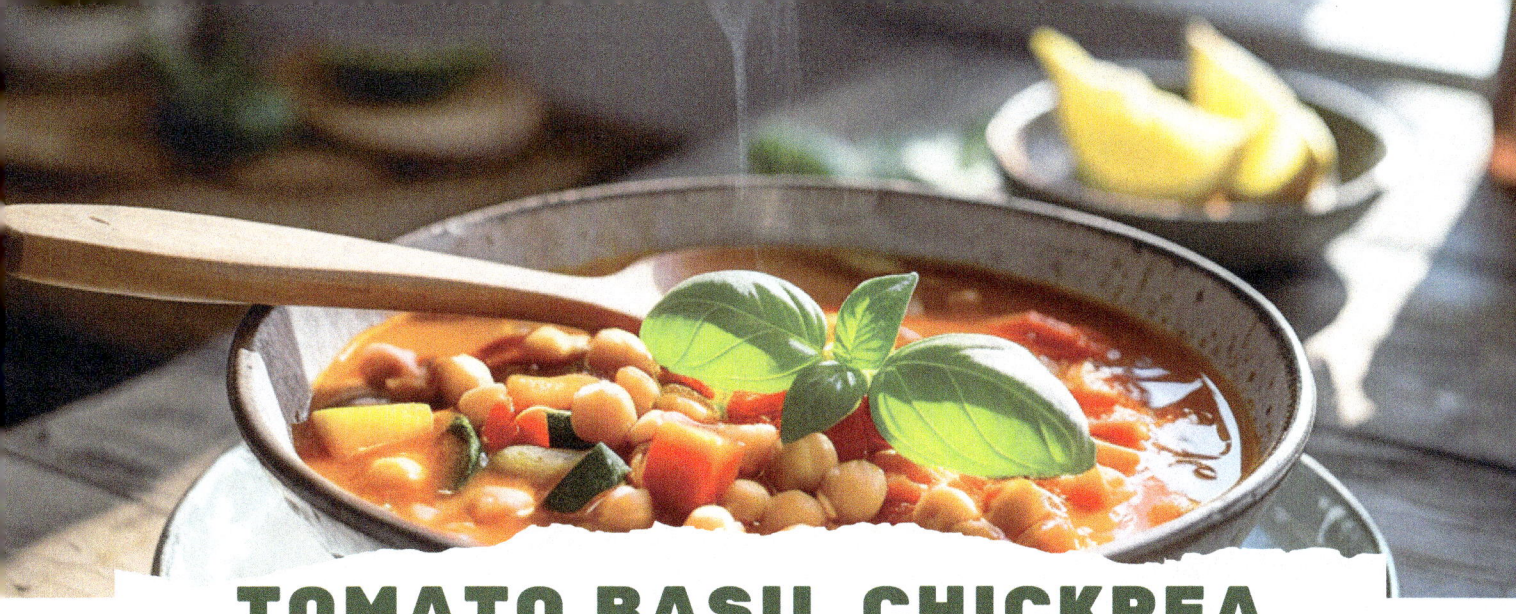

TOMATO BASIL CHICKPEA STEW

Servings: 4   **Total Time:** 30 Min

Calories: 280 | **Protein:** 10g | **Carbohydrates:** 45g | **Fat:** 7g

Ingredients

- 2 tbsp olive oil
- 1 medium onion, chopped
- 3 garlic cloves, minced
- 1 large carrot, diced
- 1 zucchini, diced
- 2 cans (15 oz) chickpeas, drained and rinsed
- 1 can (14.5 oz) diced tomatoes
- 1 cup vegetable broth
- 1 tsp dried basil
- 1/2 tsp dried oregano
- Salt and pepper, to taste
- 1/4 cup fresh basil leaves, chopped
- 1 tbsp lemon juice

Directions

- Heat olive oil in a large pot over medium heat.
- Add the chopped onion and sauté for 3-4 minutes until softened.
- Add the garlic, diced carrot, and zucchini to the pot. Cook for 5 minutes, stirring occasionally.
- Stir in the chickpeas, diced tomatoes (with juices), vegetable broth, basil, oregano, salt, and pepper.
- Bring the stew to a boil, then reduce the heat to low. Let it simmer for 15-20 minutes, stirring occasionally, until the vegetables are tender and the flavors are well blended.
- Stir in the fresh basil leaves and cook for another 2 minutes.
- Add lemon juice for a burst of freshness (optional).
- Serve hot, and enjoy your hearty, warming stew!

Tips

- Make it spicy: Add a pinch of red pepper flakes for a bit of heat.
- Blend for creaminess: If you prefer a smoother texture, blend half of the stew with an immersion blender before adding the fresh basil.
- Serve with crusty bread: This stew pairs perfectly with warm, crusty whole-grain bread for a complete meal.
- Meal prep: This stew stores well in the fridge for up to 3 days or can be frozen for up to 1 month.

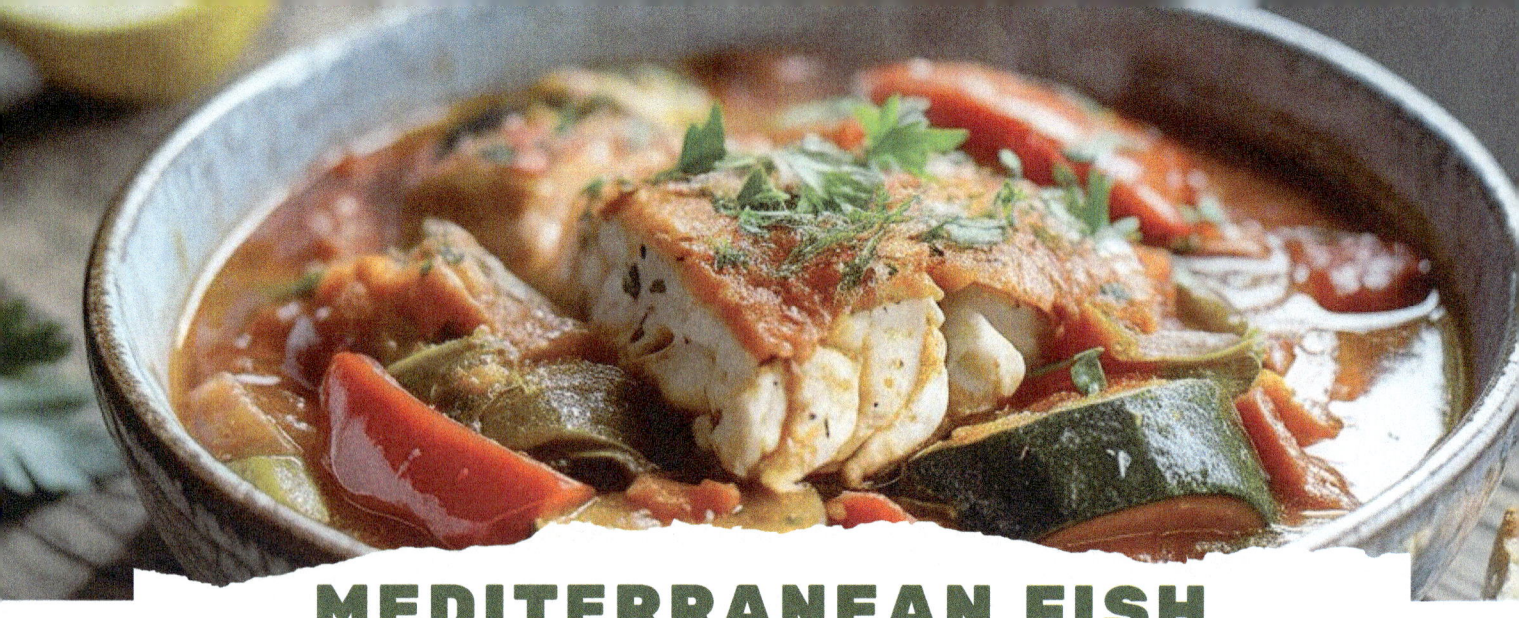

MEDITERRANEAN FISH STEW

Servings: 4 **Total Time:** 40 Min

Calories: 230 | **Protein:** 28g | **Fat:** 7g | **Carbohydrates:** 14g

Ingredients

- 1 tablespoon extra-virgin olive oil
- 1 medium onion, chopped
- 2 garlic cloves, minced
- 1 red bell pepper, diced
- 1 zucchini, sliced
- 1 can (14.5 oz) diced tomatoes (no salt added)
- 3 cups low-sodium vegetable or fish broth
- 1 teaspoon smoked paprika
- ½ teaspoon dried thyme
- ¼ teaspoon crushed red pepper flakes (optional)
- Salt and black pepper to taste
- 1½ pounds white fish fillets (such as cod or halibut), cut into chunks
- Juice of ½ lemon
- Fresh parsley, chopped (for garnish)

Directions

- In a large pot, heat the olive oil over medium heat. Add the chopped onion and sauté for 3–4 minutes, until softened.
- Add garlic, bell pepper, and zucchini. Cook for another 5 minutes, stirring occasionally.
- Stir in the diced tomatoes, broth, paprika, thyme, and crushed red pepper flakes. Bring to a gentle boil.
- Reduce heat to low and simmer uncovered for 15 minutes, allowing the flavors to blend.
- Add the fish chunks to the pot. Simmer for another 8–10 minutes, or until the fish is cooked through and flakes easily with a fork.
- Squeeze in the lemon juice and stir gently.
- Ladle into bowls, garnish with fresh parsley, and serve warm.

Tips

- Use firm white fish like cod, halibut, or sea bass so it holds together well in the stew.
- Add a handful of spinach or kale at the end for extra nutrients.
- Serve with a slice of crusty whole-grain bread or over brown rice for a heartier meal.
- Store leftovers in an airtight container for up to 2 days in the refrigerator.

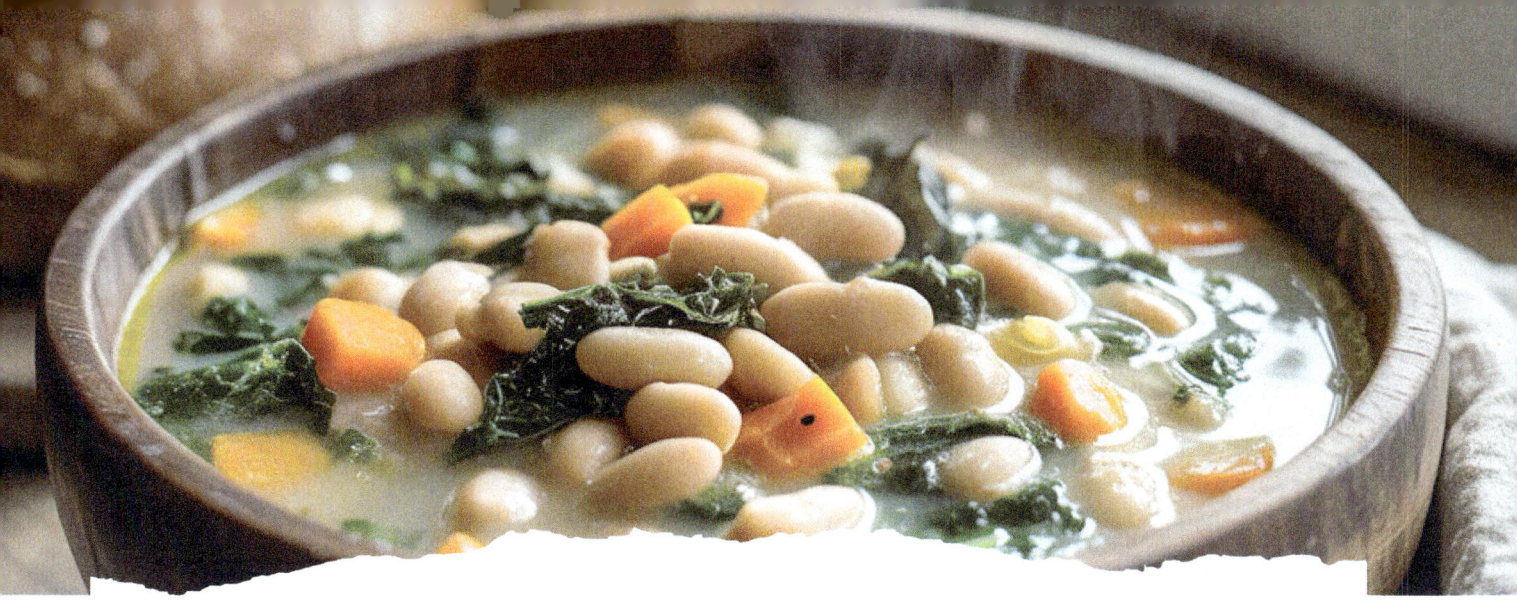

WHITE BEAN AND KALE SOUP

Servings: 4　　**Total Time:** 35 Min

Calories: 190 | **Protein:** 9 | **Fat:** 5g | **Carbohydrates:** 28g

Ingredients

- 1 tablespoon extra-virgin olive oil
- 1 small yellow onion, chopped
- 2 garlic cloves, minced
- 2 carrots, peeled and diced
- 2 celery stalks, diced
- 1 teaspoon dried thyme
- 1 teaspoon dried oregano
- 1/2 teaspoon crushed red pepper flakes (optional)
- 1 can (15 oz) white beans (cannellini or great northern), drained and rinsed
- 4 cups low-sodium vegetable broth
- 2 cups chopped fresh kale (stems removed)
- Salt and black pepper to taste
- Juice of 1/2 lemon (optional, for brightness)

Directions

- Heat olive oil in a large pot over medium heat.
- Add chopped onion, carrots, and celery. Sauté for 5–7 minutes until softened.
- Stir in garlic, thyme, oregano, and red pepper flakes. Cook for another minute.
- Add white beans and vegetable broth. Bring to a boil, then reduce heat and simmer for 15 minutes.
- Stir in chopped kale and cook for another 5 minutes, until kale is tender.
- Season with salt, pepper, and a splash of lemon juice if desired.
- Serve warm with whole grain bread or a sprinkle of grated Parmesan (optional).

Tips

- For added protein, stir in cooked shredded chicken or diced turkey.
- Swap kale with spinach or Swiss chard if preferred.
- Use an immersion blender to partially puree the soup for a creamier texture.
- Make it ahead – this soup stores well in the fridge for up to 4 days or can be frozen for 1 month.

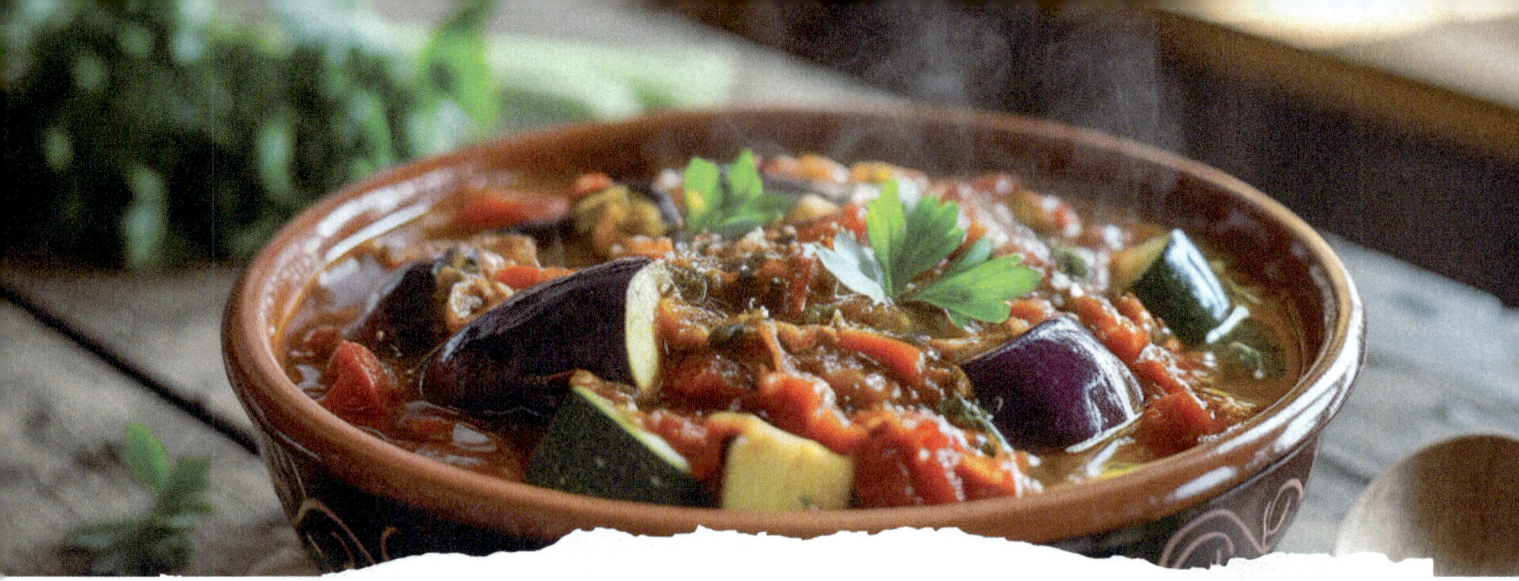

EGGPLANT AND ZUCCHINI STEW

Servings: 4 **Total Time:** 45 Min

Calories: 130 | **Protein:** 3 | **Fat:** 17g | **Carbohydrates:** 7g

Ingredients

- 1 medium eggplant, diced
- 2 medium zucchinis, sliced
- 1 large onion, chopped
- 2 garlic cloves, minced
- 1 can (14 oz) diced tomatoes (no salt added)
- 2 tbsp extra virgin olive oil
- 1 tsp dried oregano
- ½ tsp ground cumin (optional)
- Salt and pepper, to taste
- 1 cup low-sodium vegetable broth
- Fresh parsley for garnish

Directions

- Heat olive oil in a large pot over medium heat. Add the chopped onion and sauté for 3–4 minutes until soft.
- Add garlic and cook for 1 more minute until fragrant.
- Stir in the diced eggplant and cook for 5–7 minutes, stirring occasionally, until slightly tender.
- Add the zucchini, diced tomatoes, oregano, cumin (if using), salt, and pepper. Stir well to combine.
- Pour in the vegetable broth. Cover and simmer over low heat for 20–25 minutes, until all vegetables are soft and flavors are blended.
- Taste and adjust seasoning if needed. Garnish with fresh parsley before serving.

Tips

- For a heartier stew, serve over brown rice, quinoa, or couscous.
- Add chickpeas or white beans for extra protein.
- This stew tastes even better the next day as the flavors deepen – perfect for meal prep!

SPICED CARROT AND RED LENTIL SOUP

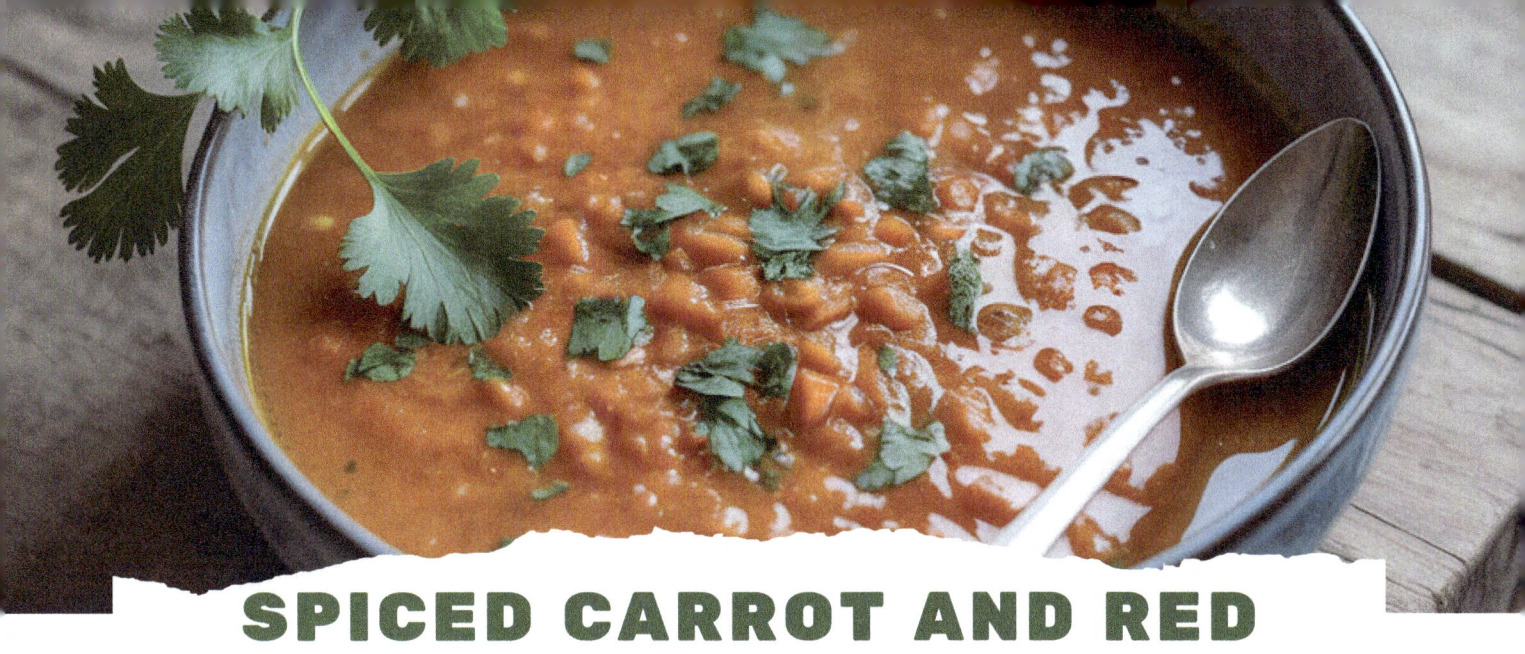

Servings: 4 | **Total Time:** 35 Min

Calories: 180 | **Protein:** 9g | **Fat:** 5g | **Carbohydrates:** 26g

Ingredients

- 1 tablespoon olive oil
- 1 small onion, chopped
- 2 garlic cloves, minced
- 1 teaspoon ground cumin
- 1/2 teaspoon ground coriander
- 1/4 teaspoon ground turmeric
- 4 medium carrots, peeled and diced
- 3/4 cup red lentils, rinsed
- 4 cups low-sodium vegetable broth
- Salt and black pepper to taste
- Juice of 1/2 lemon (optional)
- Fresh parsley or cilantro, for garnish (optional)

Directions

- Heat olive oil in a large pot over medium heat. Add chopped onion and cook for 3–4 minutes until softened.
- Stir in garlic, cumin, coriander, and turmeric. Cook for 1 minute until fragrant.
- Add diced carrots and cook for another 3–4 minutes, stirring occasionally.
- Pour in the rinsed red lentils and vegetable broth. Stir well.
- Bring to a boil, then reduce heat, cover, and simmer for 20–25 minutes, or until carrots and lentils are soft.
- Use an immersion blender to blend the soup until smooth, or leave it slightly chunky if preferred.
- Season with salt, pepper, and a squeeze of lemon juice if desired.
- Garnish with chopped fresh herbs before serving.

Tips

- For added creaminess, stir in a spoonful of Greek yogurt before serving.
- This soup freezes well – store in portions for up to 3 months.
- Serve with whole grain pita or a side salad for a heartier meal.
- Add a pinch of chili flakes if you prefer a little heat.

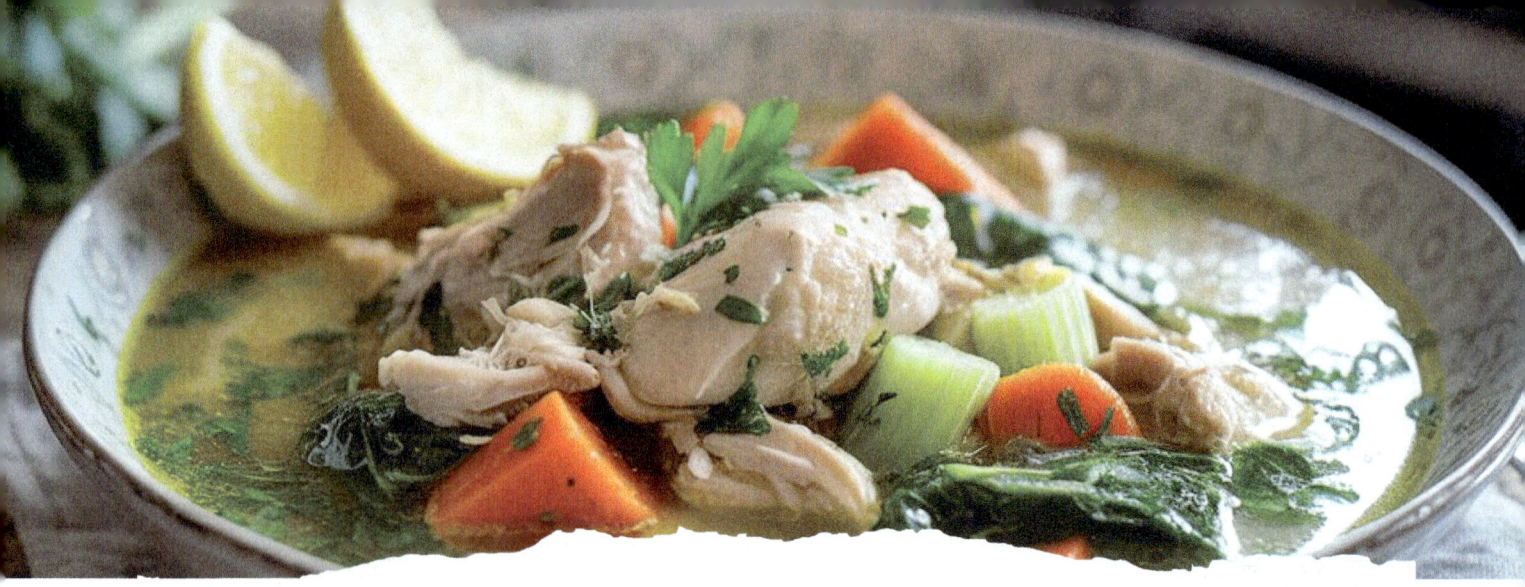

LEMON GARLIC CHICKEN STEW

Servings: 4 | **Total Time:** 45 Min

Calories: 280 | **Protein:** 28g | **Carbohydrates:** 12g | **Fat:** 14g

Ingredients

- 1 lb (450g) boneless, skinless chicken thighs, cut into chunks
- 2 tablespoons olive oil
- 1 medium onion, chopped
- 4 garlic cloves, minced
- 2 carrots, sliced
- 2 celery stalks, chopped
- 1 teaspoon dried oregano
- 1/2 teaspoon ground black pepper
- Salt to taste
- Juice of 1 lemon
- 4 cups low-sodium chicken broth
- 1 cup baby spinach
- Fresh parsley, chopped (for garnish)

Directions

- Heat olive oil in a large pot over medium heat.
- Add chopped onion and sauté for 2–3 minutes until translucent.
- Stir in garlic and cook for 30 seconds until fragrant.
- Add chicken pieces and cook until lightly browned on all sides, about 5–7 minutes.
- Add carrots, celery, oregano, black pepper, and a pinch of salt. Stir well.
- Pour in chicken broth and bring to a boil.
- Reduce heat and let the stew simmer for 25 minutes, or until chicken is fully cooked and vegetables are tender.
- Stir in lemon juice and baby spinach (if using), and cook for 2 more minutes.
- Taste and adjust seasoning if needed.
- Serve hot, garnished with chopped fresh parsley.

Tips

- For extra lemon flavor, add a bit of lemon zest along with the juice.
- This stew pairs wonderfully with a slice of whole-grain bread or brown rice.
- Store leftovers in the fridge for up to 3 days – it tastes even better the next day!

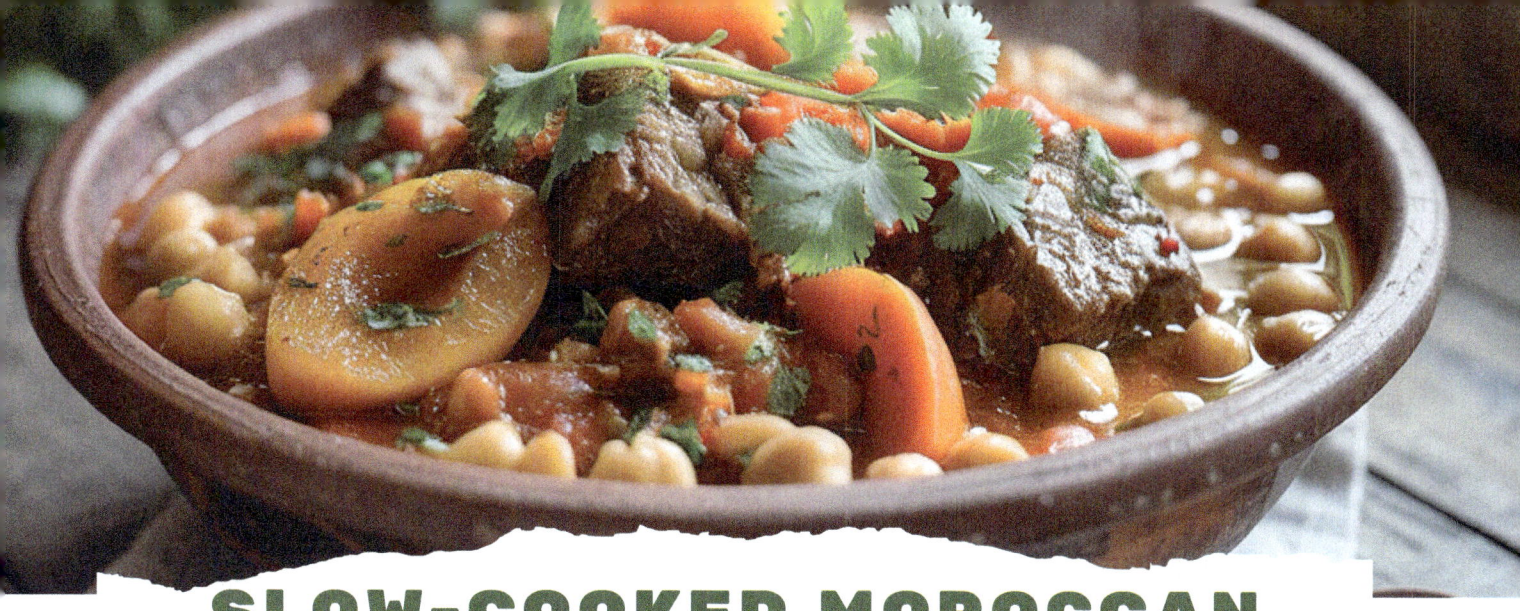

SLOW-COOKED MOROCCAN LAMB STEW

Servings: 4   **Total Time:** 45 Min

Calories: 430 | **Protein:** 32g | **Fat:** 18g | **Carbohydrates:** 34g

Ingredients

- 1½ lbs (700g) lamb shoulder, trimmed and cut into chunks
- 1 tbsp olive oil
- 1 onion, chopped
- 2 cloves garlic, minced
- 1 tsp ground cumin
- 1 tsp ground cinnamon
- ½ tsp ground ginger
- ½ tsp paprika
- ¼ tsp ground turmeric
- 1 (14 oz) can diced tomatoes
- 1½ cups low-sodium chicken broth
- 1 tbsp tomato paste
- 1 large carrot, peeled and sliced
- ½ cup dried apricots, chopped
- 1 (15 oz) can chickpeas, drained and rinsed
- Salt and black pepper to taste
- Fresh cilantro or parsley, chopped (for garnish)

Directions

- Brown the lamb: Heat olive oil in a large skillet over medium-high heat. Add lamb and brown on all sides (about 5–6 minutes). Transfer to your slow cooker.
- Sauté aromatics: In the same pan, add chopped onion and cook for 3–4 minutes until softened. Stir in garlic, cumin, cinnamon, ginger, paprika, and turmeric. Cook for 1 minute, stirring constantly.
- Combine in slow cooker: Add the onion-spice mixture to the slow cooker along with diced tomatoes, chicken broth, tomato paste, carrots, and apricots. Stir to combine.
- Cook: Cover and cook on low for 6 hours or high for 3½–4 hours, until the lamb is tender.
- Add chickpeas: Stir in chickpeas 30 minutes before serving.
- Finish: Season with salt and pepper to taste. Garnish with fresh herbs before serving.

Tips

- For deeper flavor, marinate the lamb overnight in olive oil, garlic, and spices.
- This stew pairs wonderfully with whole wheat couscous, quinoa, or crusty whole grain bread.
- Leftovers taste even better the next day – store in an airtight container in the fridge for up to 3 days or freeze for up to 2 months.

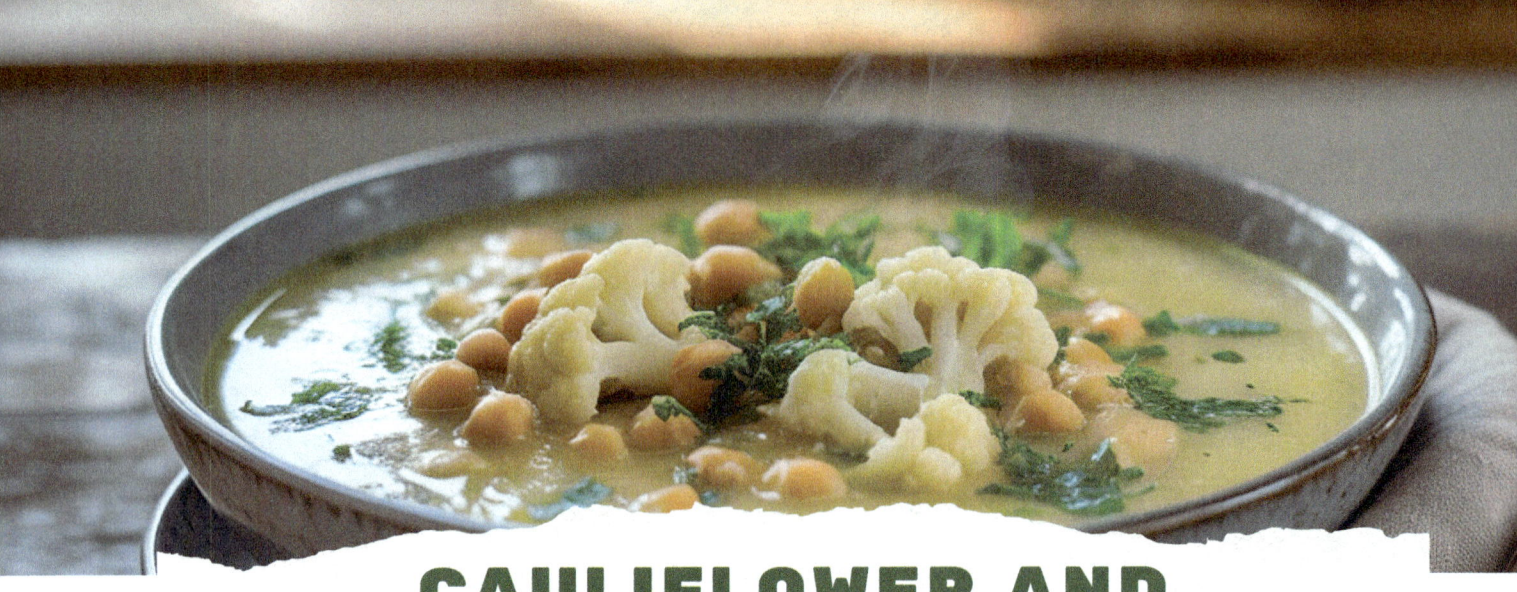

CAULIFLOWER AND CHICKPEA SOUP

Servings: 4   **Total Time:** 35 Min

Calories: 180 | **Protein:** 8g | **Carbohydrates:** 25g | **Fat:** 5g

Ingredients

- 1 tablespoon extra-virgin olive oil
- 1 small onion, chopped
- 2 garlic cloves, minced
- 1 teaspoon ground cumin
- 1/2 teaspoon ground turmeric
- 1 head cauliflower, cut into florets
- 1 (15 oz) can chickpeas, drained and rinsed
- 4 cups low-sodium vegetable broth
- Salt and pepper to taste
- Juice of 1/2 lemon
- Fresh parsley for garnish

Directions

- In a large pot, heat olive oil over medium heat. Add chopped onion and sauté for 4–5 minutes until soft.
- Add garlic, cumin, and turmeric. Cook for another 1 minute until fragrant.
- Stir in the cauliflower florets and chickpeas. Mix well to coat with the spices.
- Pour in the vegetable broth. Bring to a boil, then reduce heat and simmer uncovered for 20 minutes, or until cauliflower is tender.
- Use an immersion blender to partially puree the soup for a creamy texture, leaving some chunks for bite.
- Stir in lemon juice and season with salt and pepper to taste.
- Ladle into bowls, garnish with parsley if desired, and serve warm.

Tips

- Add a pinch of red pepper flakes for a spicy kick.
- This soup stores well in the fridge for up to 3 days – perfect for meal prep.
- For extra creaminess, stir in a spoonful of Greek yogurt before serving.

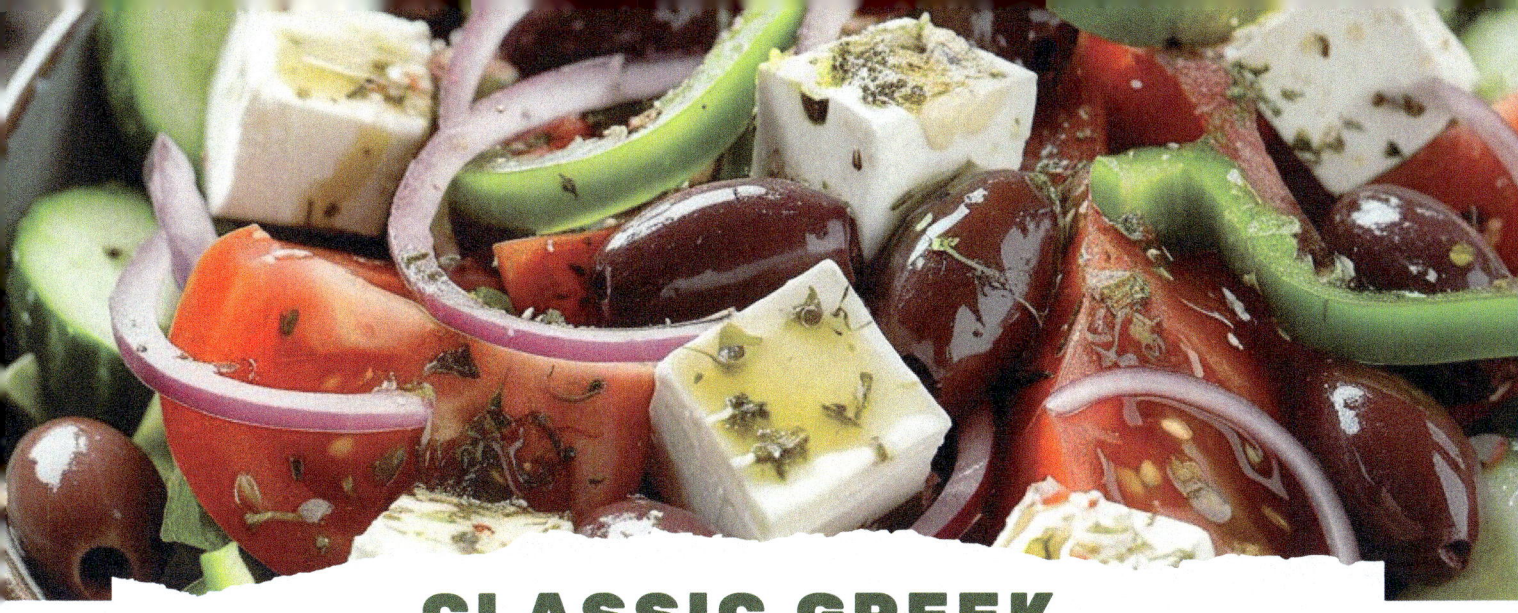

CLASSIC GREEK SALAD

Servings: 4   **Total Time:** 15 Min

Calories: 180 | **Protein:** 5g | **Fat:** 15g | **Carbohydrates:** 8g

Ingredients

- 4 medium ripe tomatoes, cut into wedges
- 1 cucumber, peeled and sliced
- 1 small red onion, thinly sliced
- 1 green bell pepper, sliced
- 1/2 cup Kalamata olives
- 1/2 cup feta cheese, cut into cubes or crumbled
- 2 tbsp extra virgin olive oil
- 1 tbsp red wine vinegar
- 1 tsp dried oregano
- Salt and black pepper to taste

Directions

- In a large salad bowl, combine the tomatoes, cucumber, red onion, and green bell pepper.
- Add the olives and feta cheese on top.
- In a small bowl, whisk together the olive oil, red wine vinegar, oregano, salt, and pepper.
- Drizzle the dressing over the salad and gently toss to combine.
- Serve immediately or chill for 10–15 minutes for enhanced flavor.

Tips

- Use high-quality olive oil and fresh vegetables for best flavor.
- For a heartier salad, add cooked quinoa or chickpeas.
- You can replace red wine vinegar with lemon juice for a citrusy twist.

QUINOA AND ROASTED VEGETABLE SALAD

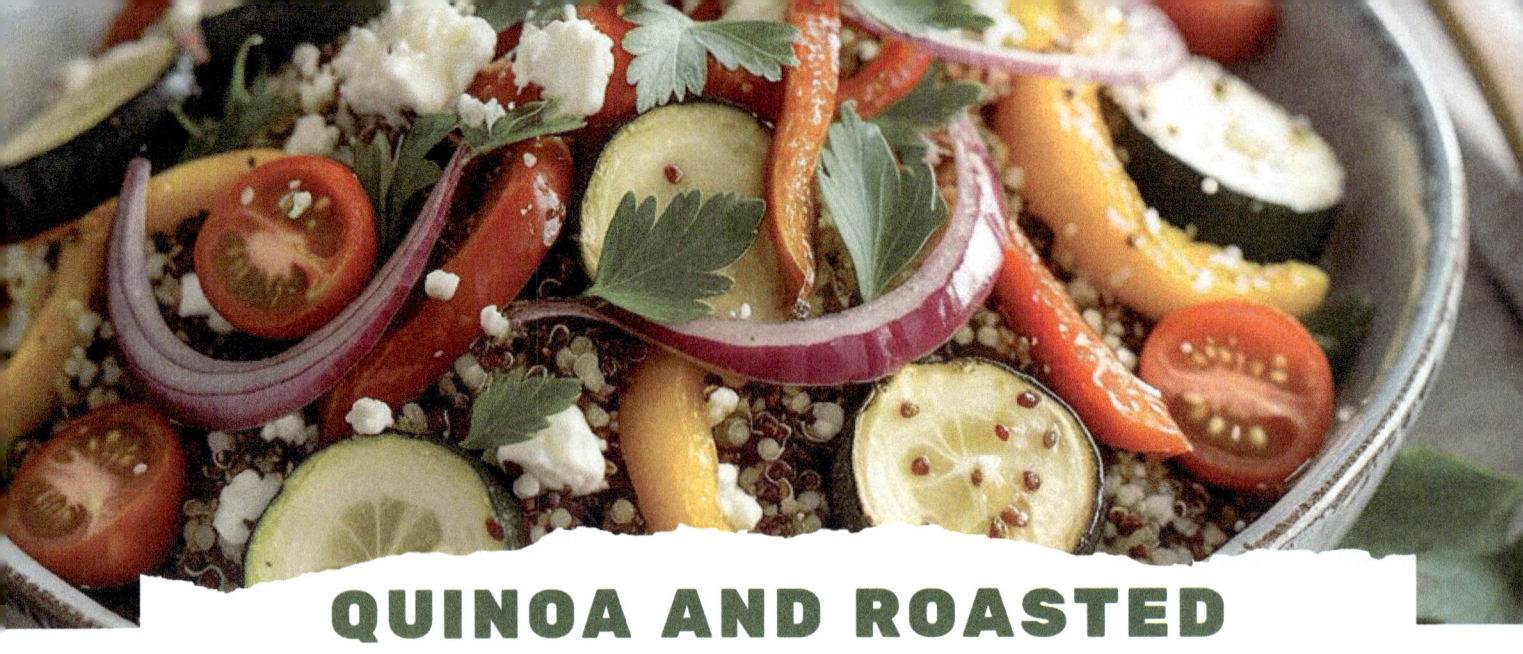

Servings: 4 | **Total Time:** 40 Min

Calories: ~280 | **Protein:** 8g | **Carbohydrates:** 35g | **Fat:** 12g

Ingredients

- 1 cup quinoa (rinsed)
- 2 cups water or low-sodium vegetable broth
- 1 zucchini, chopped
- 1 red bell pepper, chopped
- 1 yellow bell pepper, chopped
- 1 small red onion, chopped
- 1 cup cherry tomatoes, halved
- 2 tablespoons extra-virgin olive oil
- 1 teaspoon dried oregano
- Salt and black pepper to taste
- Juice of 1 lemon
- 2 tablespoons chopped fresh parsley or basil
- Optional: crumbled feta cheese (¼ cup)

Directions

- Preheat the oven to 400°F (200°C).
- Place the chopped zucchini, bell peppers, onion, and cherry tomatoes on a baking sheet. Drizzle with 1 tablespoon of olive oil, sprinkle with oregano, salt, and pepper. Toss to coat evenly.
- Roast the vegetables in the oven for 20–25 minutes or until tender and slightly charred.
- Meanwhile, cook the quinoa: In a medium pot, bring 2 cups of water or broth to a boil. Add quinoa, reduce heat to low, cover, and simmer for 15 minutes or until liquid is absorbed. Fluff with a fork.
- Let the quinoa and vegetables cool slightly.
- In a large bowl, combine quinoa and roasted vegetables. Drizzle with remaining olive oil and lemon juice. Toss gently.
- Sprinkle with fresh parsley (or basil) and feta if using. Serve warm or chilled.

Tips

- Add a handful of arugula or spinach for extra greens.
- Store leftovers in the fridge for up to 3 days — it tastes great cold.
- Swap quinoa with bulgur or couscous for variety.
- For added protein, toss in chickpeas or grilled chicken.

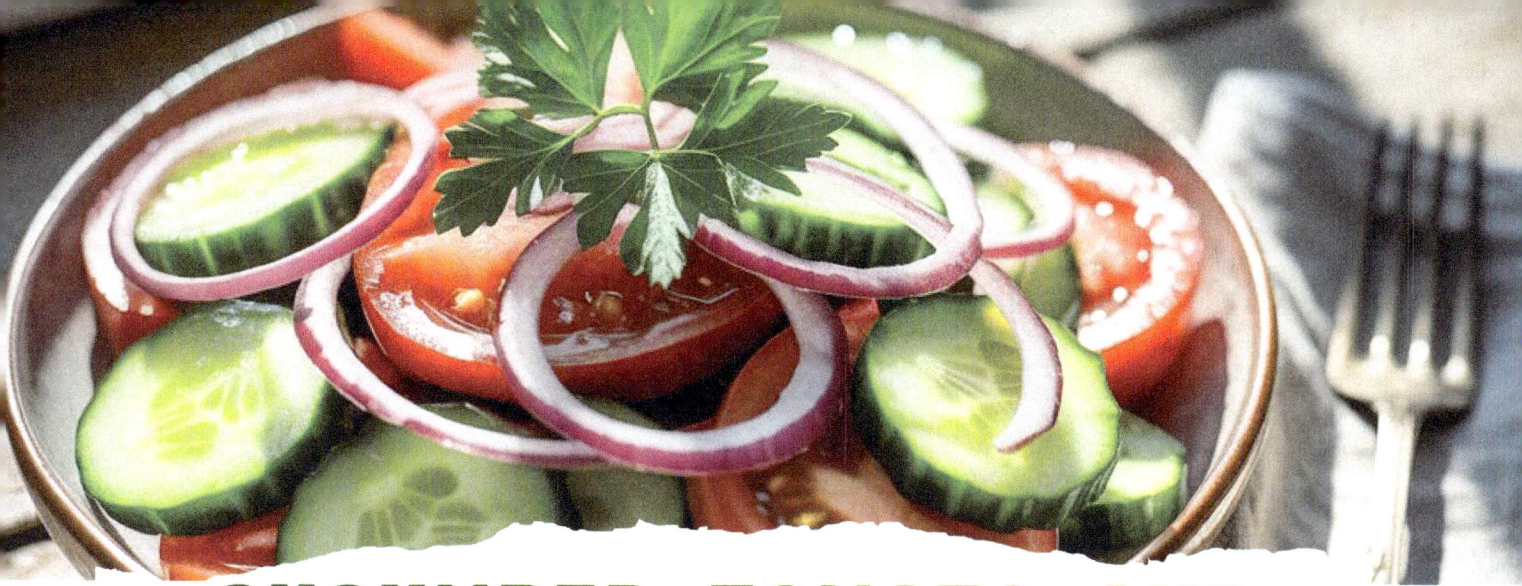

CUCUMBER, TOMATO, AND RED ONION SALAD

Servings: 4   **Total Time:** 10 Min

Calories: 90 | **Fat:** 7g | **Carbohydrates:** 7g | **Protein:** 1g

Ingredients

- 2 medium cucumbers, thinly sliced
- 2 large tomatoes, chopped
- 1 small red onion, thinly sliced
- 2 tablespoons extra-virgin olive oil
- 1 tablespoon red wine vinegar or lemon juice
- Salt and black pepper to taste
- 1 tablespoon chopped fresh parsley (optional)
- ½ teaspoon dried oregano (optional)

Directions

- In a large bowl, combine the sliced cucumbers, chopped tomatoes, and red onion.
- In a small bowl, whisk together the olive oil, vinegar or lemon juice, salt, pepper, and optional oregano.
- Pour the dressing over the vegetables and toss gently to coat.
- Garnish with fresh parsley if desired.
- Serve immediately or refrigerate for 10–15 minutes to let the flavors blend.

Tips

- For extra flavor, add crumbled feta cheese or sliced olives.
- To mellow the sharpness of the onion, soak slices in cold water for 5–10 minutes before adding.
- This salad pairs perfectly with grilled fish or chicken for a light Mediterranean meal.

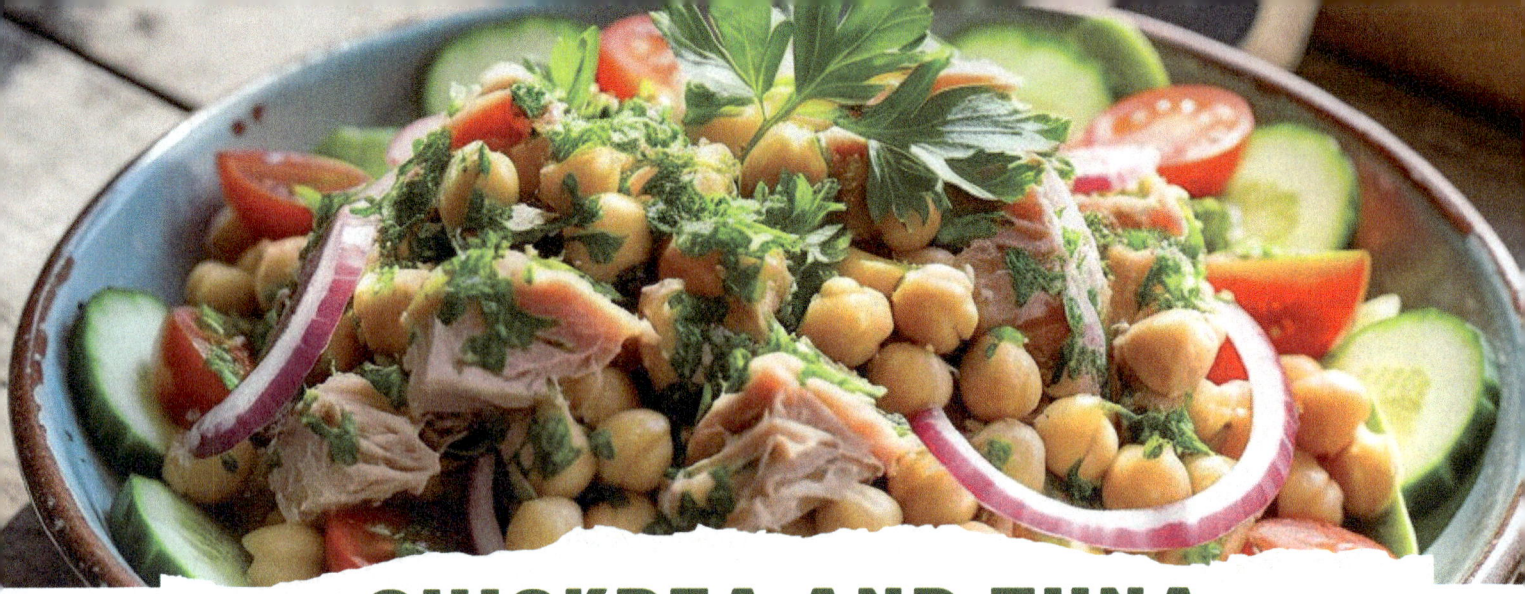

CHICKPEA AND TUNA SALAD

Servings: 2 **Total Time:** 10 Min

Calories: 310 | **Protein:** 21g | **Carbohydrates:** 22g | **Fat:** 16g

Ingredients

- 1 can (15 oz) chickpeas, drained and rinsed
- 1 can (5 oz) tuna in olive oil, drained
- 1 small red onion, thinly sliced
- 1 small cucumber, diced
- 1 cup cherry tomatoes, halved
- 2 tablespoons fresh parsley, chopped
- 2 tablespoons extra-virgin olive oil
- Juice of 1 lemon
- Salt and pepper to taste

Directions

- In a large bowl, combine the chickpeas, tuna, red onion, cucumber, and cherry tomatoes.
- Add the chopped parsley and gently toss to mix.
- In a small bowl, whisk together olive oil, lemon juice, salt, and pepper.
- Pour the dressing over the salad and toss until well coated.
- Serve immediately or chill for 15 minutes for enhanced flavor.

Tips

- For extra flavor, add a pinch of oregano or a few capers.
- Use canned salmon or grilled chicken as an alternative to tuna.
- Pairs well with whole grain pita or served over mixed greens for a light meal.

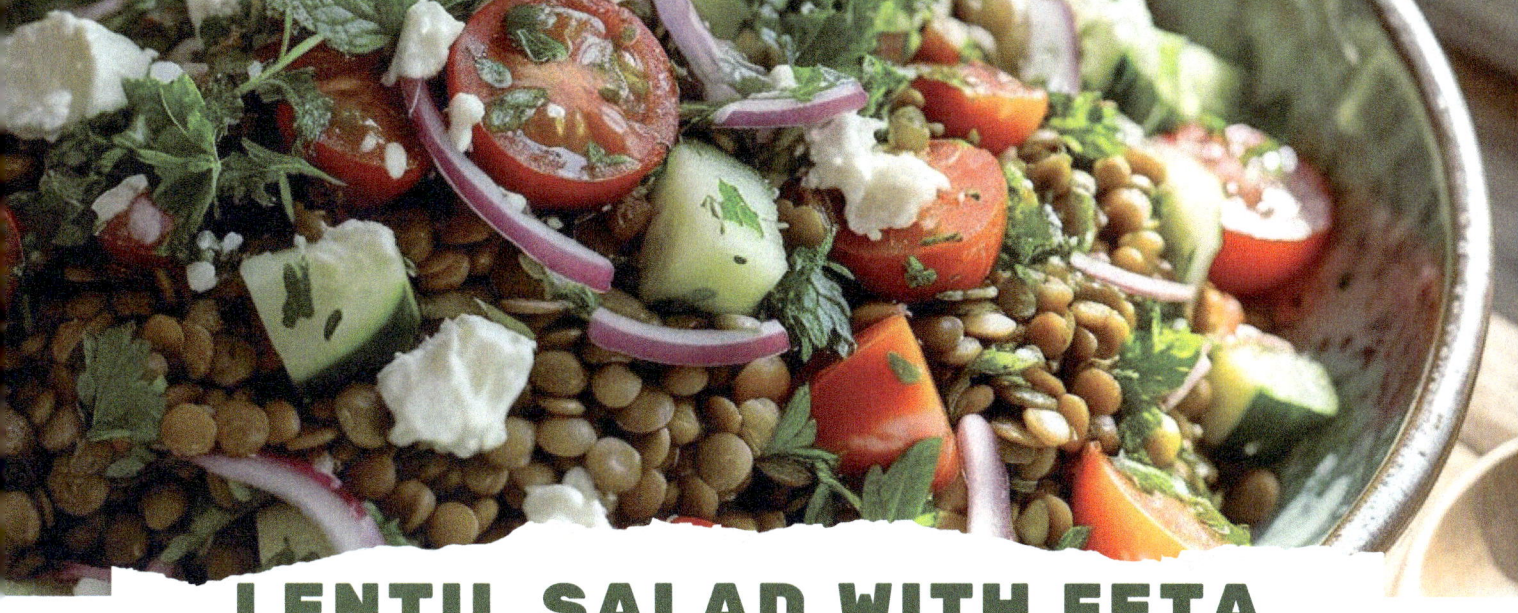

LENTIL SALAD WITH FETA AND HERBS

Servings: 4 | **Total Time:** 30 Min

Calories: 260 | **Protein:** 12g | **Carbohydrates:** 30g | **Fat:** 10g

Ingredients

- 1 cup dried green or brown lentils (or 2 ½ cups cooked lentils)
- 1 bay leaf (optional, for cooking lentils)
- ½ small red onion, finely diced
- ½ cup fresh parsley, chopped
- 2 tablespoons fresh mint, chopped
- 1 cup cherry tomatoes, halved
- ½ cucumber, diced
- ½ cup crumbled feta cheese
- 2 tablespoons extra virgin olive oil
- 1 tablespoon lemon juice (freshly squeezed)
- Salt and black pepper to taste

Directions

- Cook the lentils: Rinse lentils thoroughly. In a medium pot, combine lentils and 3 cups of water. Add a bay leaf if desired. Bring to a boil, then reduce to a simmer. Cook for 20–25 minutes until lentils are tender but not mushy. Drain and let cool.
- Prepare vegetables and herbs: While lentils cool, chop the red onion, parsley, mint, tomatoes, and cucumber.
- Combine: In a large bowl, mix the cooled lentils with chopped vegetables and herbs.
- Dress the salad: Drizzle with olive oil and lemon juice. Add salt and pepper to taste. Gently toss to combine.
- Top with feta: Sprinkle crumbled feta cheese over the top just before serving.

Tips

- For extra flavor, add a dash of red wine vinegar or a pinch of cumin to the dressing.
- This salad keeps well in the fridge for up to 3 days – great for meal prep!
- Make it a main dish by adding grilled chicken or a boiled egg on top.
- Use canned lentils to save time (rinse and drain before using).

ARUGULA SALAD WITH PEARS AND WALNUTS

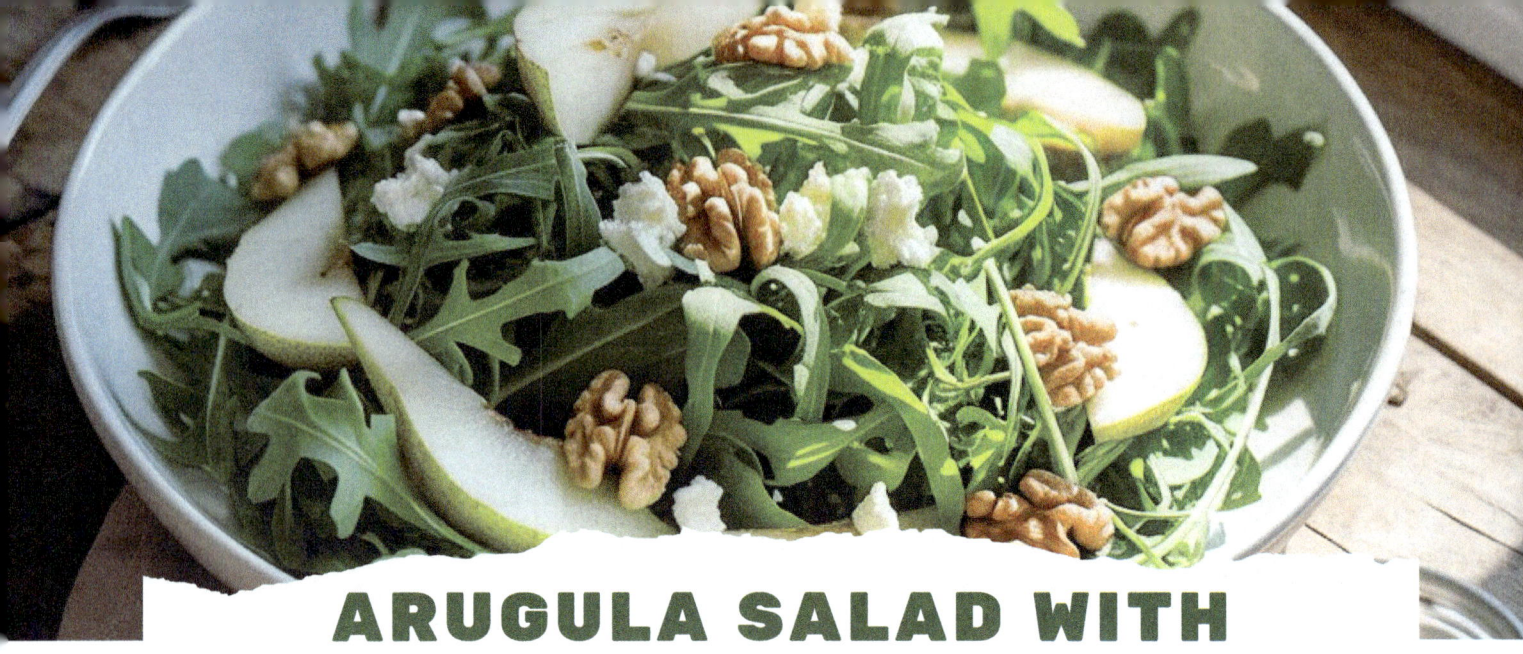

Servings: 2   **Total Time:** 10 Min

Calories: 180 | **Protein:** 3g | **Carbohydrates:** 14g | **Fat:** 14g

Ingredients

- 4 cups fresh arugula
- 1 ripe pear, thinly sliced
- ¼ cup walnut halves
- 2 tablespoons crumbled feta cheese (optional)
- 1 tablespoon extra-virgin olive oil
- 1 tablespoon balsamic vinegar
- Salt and black pepper to taste

Directions

- In a large bowl, add the arugula and pear slices.
- Sprinkle in the walnut halves and feta cheese if using.
- In a small bowl or jar, whisk together olive oil and balsamic vinegar.
- Drizzle the dressing over the salad.
- Gently toss to combine.
- Season with salt and pepper to taste.
- Serve immediately and enjoy fresh.

Tips

- For extra crunch, lightly toast the walnuts before adding.
- Swap pears with apples or figs for variation.
- Add grilled chicken or chickpeas to make it a complete meal.
- Use goat cheese or blue cheese for a different flavor profile.

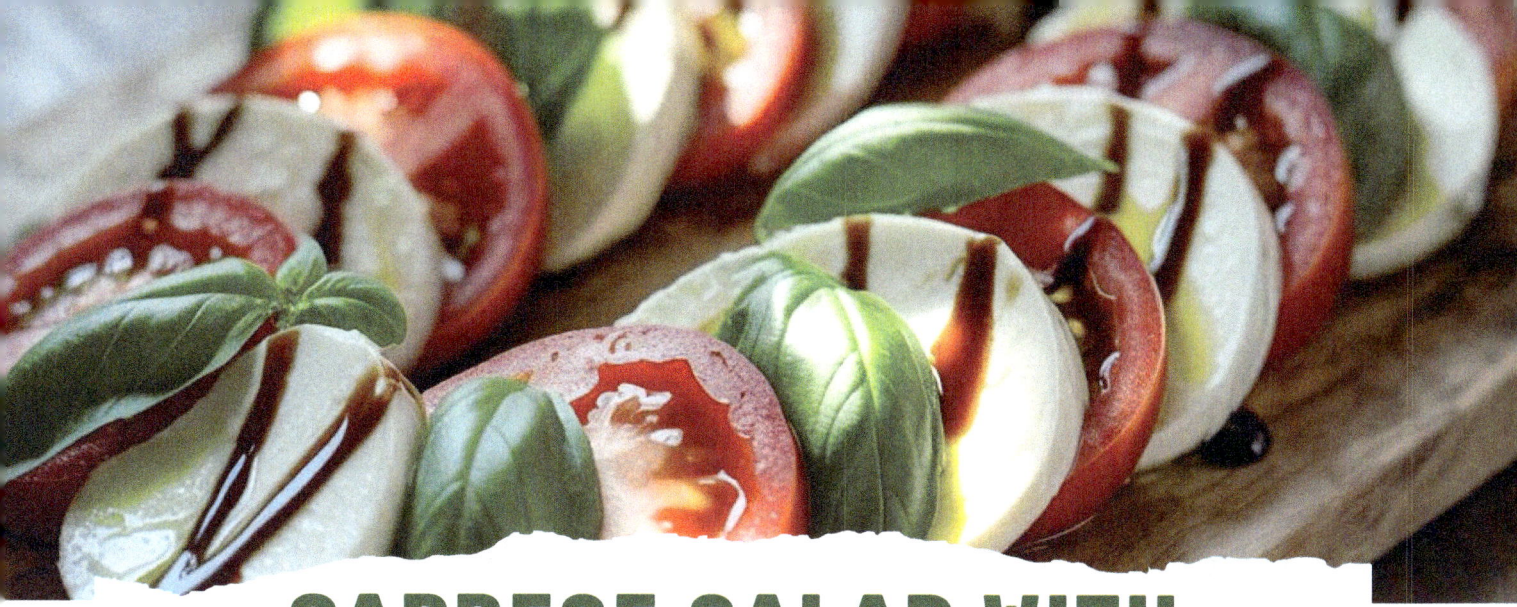

CAPRESE SALAD WITH BALSAMIC GLAZE

Servings: 2 | **Total Time:** 10 Min

Calories: 220 | **Protein:** 11g | **Fat:** 17g | **Carbohydrates:** 5g

Ingredients

- 2 medium ripe tomatoes, sliced
- 6 oz fresh mozzarella cheese, sliced
- Fresh basil leaves (about 10–12)
- 2 tablespoons balsamic glaze
- 1 tablespoon extra-virgin olive oil
- Salt and black pepper to taste

Directions

- Arrange the tomato and mozzarella slices on a plate, alternating them in a circle or line.
- Tuck whole basil leaves between each slice.
- Drizzle olive oil evenly over the salad.
- Add the balsamic glaze on top in a zigzag or circular pattern.
- Sprinkle with a pinch of salt and black pepper to taste.
- Serve immediately, or chill briefly if preferred cold.

Tips

- For best flavor, use tomatoes at room temperature.
- If balsamic glaze is unavailable, reduce balsamic vinegar over low heat until thick.
- Add a few cherry tomatoes for extra color and sweetness.
- Perfect as a light lunch, appetizer, or side dish.

MEDITERRANEAN ORZO SALAD

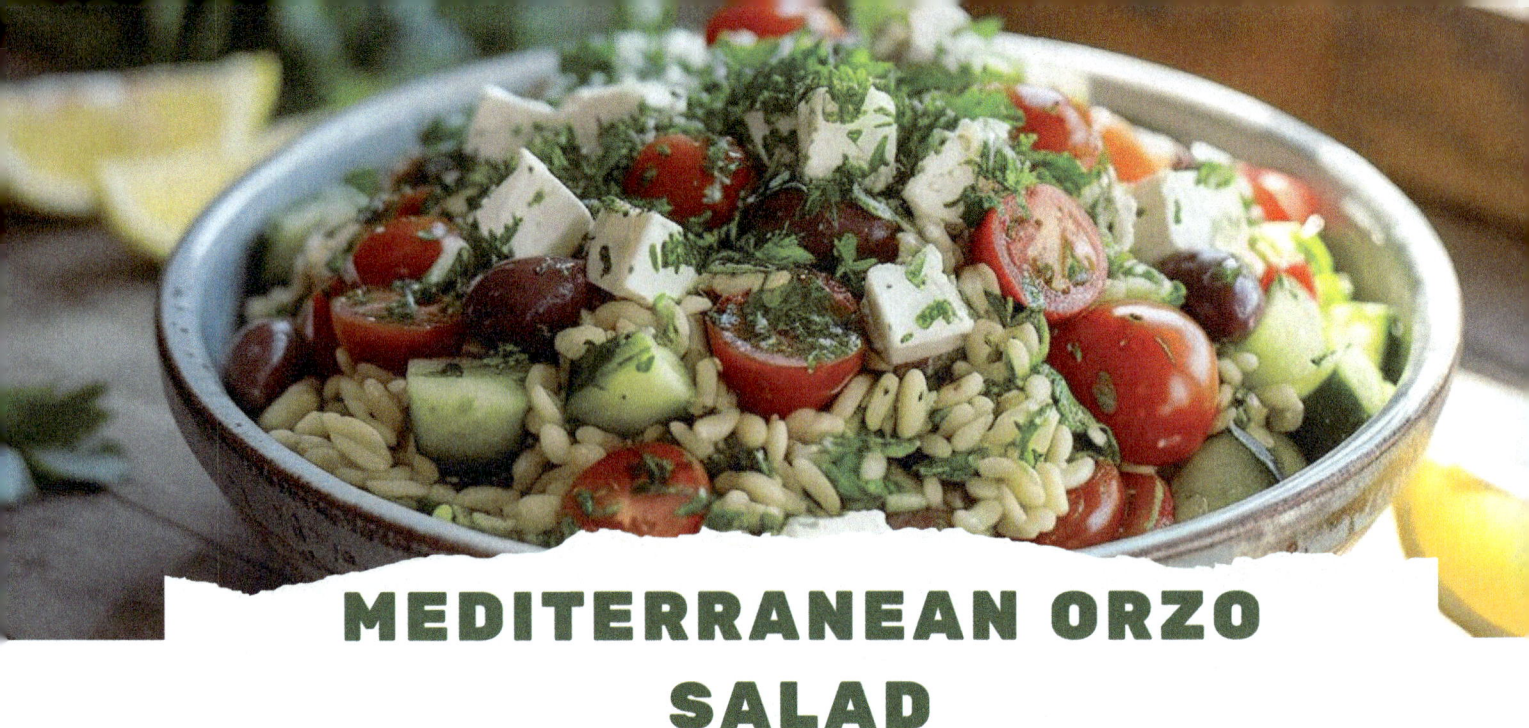

Servings: 4 | **Total Time:** 25 Min

Calories: 280 | **Protein:** 7g | **Fat:** 14g | **Carbohydrates:** 30g

Ingredients

- 1 cup orzo pasta
- 1 cup cherry tomatoes, halved
- 1/2 cup cucumber, diced
- 1/4 cup red onion, finely chopped
- 1/3 cup Kalamata olives, sliced
- 1/3 cup feta cheese, crumbled
- 2 tablespoons fresh parsley, chopped
- 2 tablespoons extra-virgin olive oil
- 1 tablespoon fresh lemon juice
- 1/2 teaspoon dried oregano
- Salt and pepper to taste

Directions

- Cook the orzo according to package instructions. Drain and rinse with cold water to cool.
- In a large bowl, combine the cooked orzo, cherry tomatoes, cucumber, red onion, olives, feta cheese, and parsley.
- In a small bowl or jar, whisk together olive oil, lemon juice, oregano, salt, and pepper.
- Pour the dressing over the salad and toss gently to coat all ingredients evenly.
- Chill for 10–15 minutes before serving, or enjoy immediately.

Tips

- You can use whole wheat orzo for added fiber and nutrition.
- Add grilled chicken or chickpeas to turn this into a hearty meal.
- Make ahead and store in the fridge for up to 3 days – great for meal prep or potlucks.

BEET AND FETA SALAD

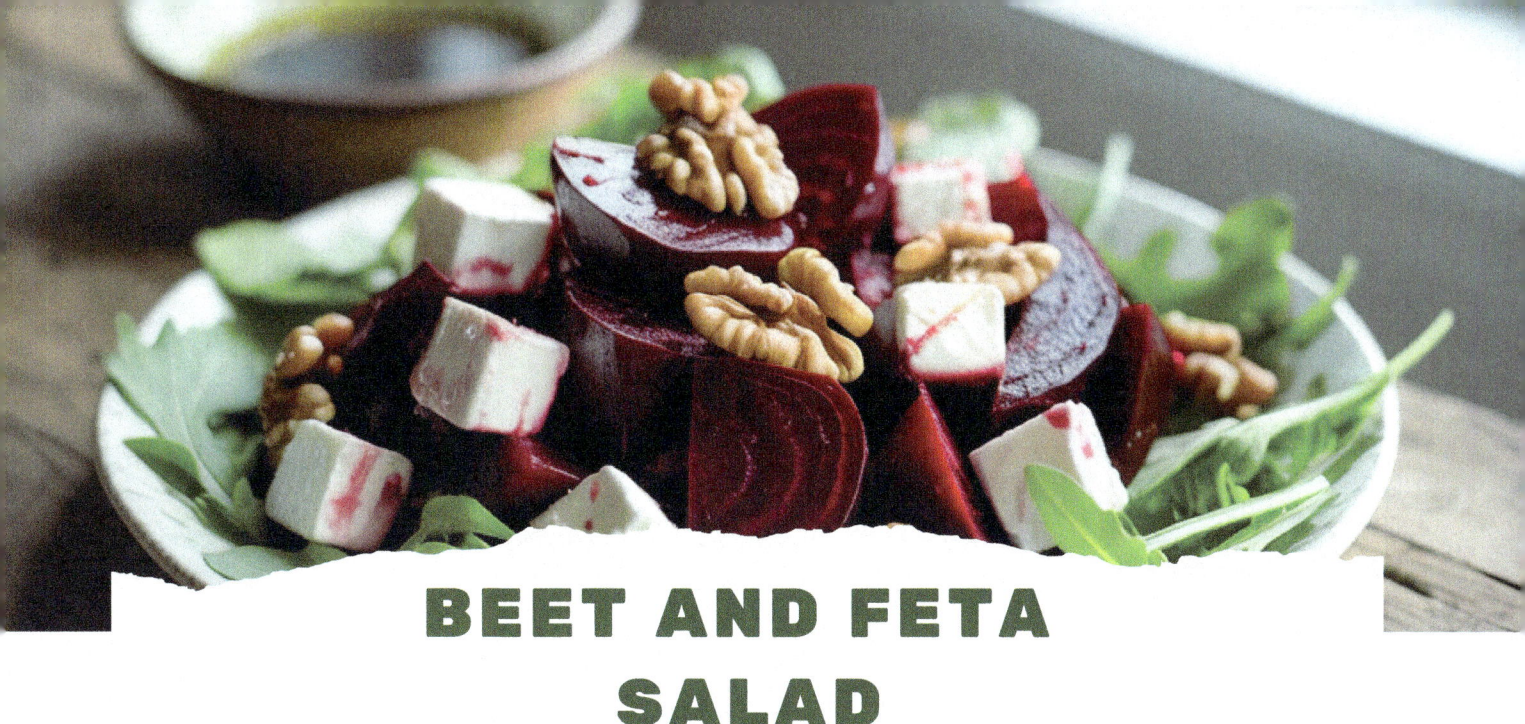

Servings: 2   **Total Time:** 35 Min

Calories: 180 | **Protein:** 5g | **Carbohydrates:** 15g | **Fat:** 12g

Ingredients

- 2 medium beets, peeled and diced
- 1 tablespoon olive oil
- 1 cup baby arugula or mixed greens
- ¼ cup crumbled feta cheese
- 2 tablespoons chopped walnuts (optional)
- 1 tablespoon balsamic vinegar
- 1 teaspoon honey (optional)
- Salt and pepper to taste

Directions

- Preheat oven to 400°F (200°C).
- Place diced beets on a baking sheet, drizzle with olive oil, and toss to coat.
- Roast for 25–30 minutes or until tender. Let cool slightly.
- In a bowl, combine greens, roasted beets, feta, and walnuts.
- In a small bowl, whisk together balsamic vinegar, honey (if using), salt, and pepper.
- Drizzle the dressing over the salad and toss gently.
- Serve fresh as a light lunch or side dish.

Tips

- Use pre-cooked beets to save time.
- Add orange slices or avocado for extra flavor and nutrients.
- For a protein boost, top with grilled chicken or chickpeas.

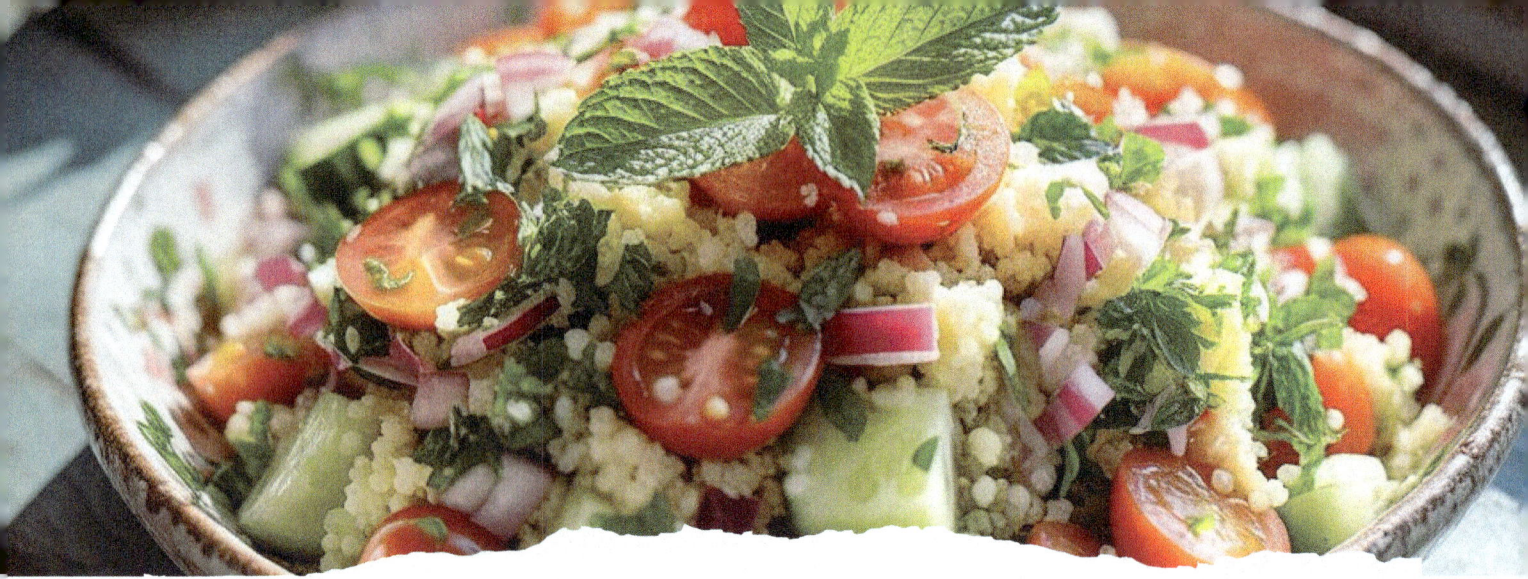

COUSCOUS SALAD WITH LEMON AND MINT

Servings: 4   **Total Time:** 20 Min

Calories: 210 | **Protein:** 5g | **Carbohydrates:** 30g | **Fat:** 8g

Ingredients

- 1 cup couscous
- 1 cup boiling water
- 2 tablespoons extra-virgin olive oil
- Juice and zest of 1 lemon
- 1/4 teaspoon salt
- 1/4 teaspoon black pepper
- 1/2 cup chopped cucumber
- 1/2 cup cherry tomatoes, halved
- 1/4 cup red onion, finely diced
- 1/4 cup chopped fresh mint
- 1/4 cup chopped fresh parsley

Directions

- In a heatproof bowl, add couscous and pour in 1 cup boiling water. Cover and let sit for 5 minutes.
- Fluff couscous with a fork to separate the grains.
- In a small bowl, whisk together olive oil, lemon juice, lemon zest, salt, and pepper.
- Add cucumber, tomatoes, red onion, mint, and parsley to the couscous.
- Pour the dressing over the salad and toss until evenly coated.
- Chill for 10–15 minutes before serving for best flavor.

Tips

- For extra protein, add chickpeas or crumbled feta cheese.
- Use whole wheat couscous for added fiber.
- This salad keeps well in the fridge for up to 2 days – great for meal prep.
- Add chopped olives or capers for a Mediterranean twist.

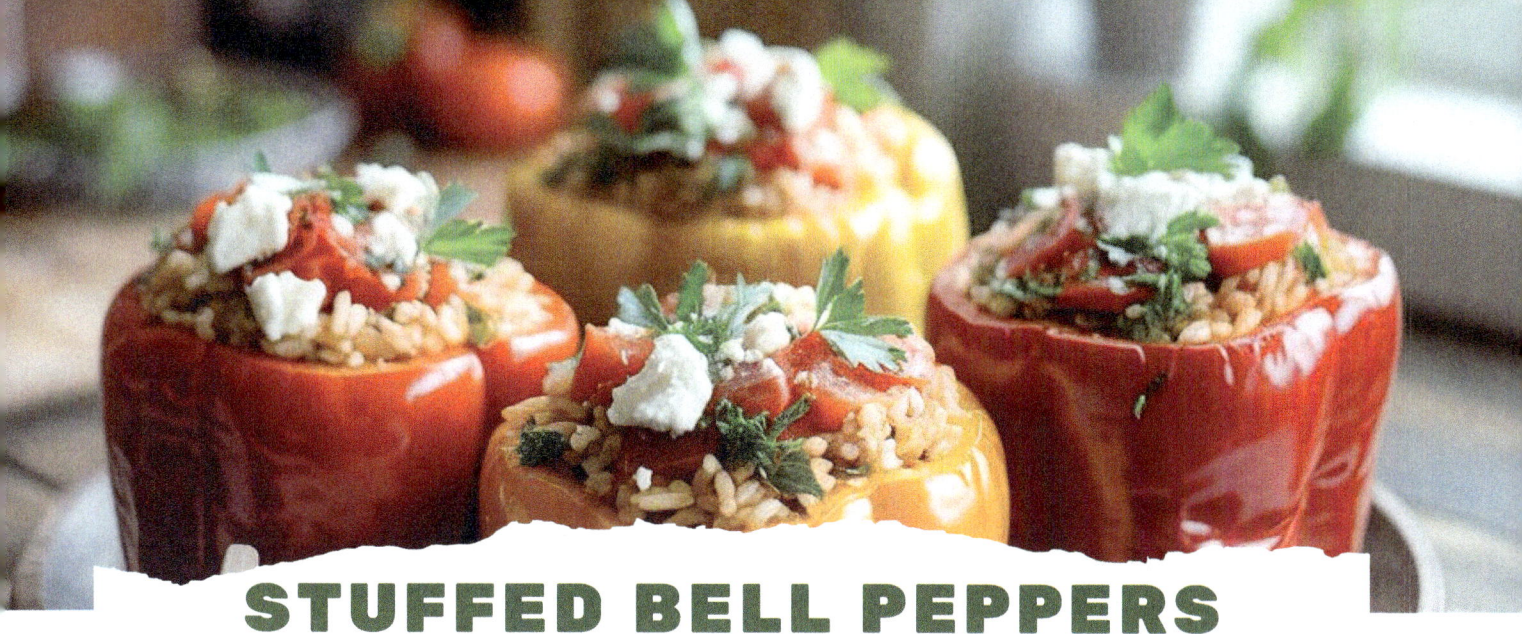

STUFFED BELL PEPPERS WITH RICE AND HERBS

Servings: 4 | **Total Time:** 50 Min

Calories: 220 | **Protein:** 5g | **Carbohydrates:** 30g | **Fat:** 9g

Ingredients

- 4 large bell peppers (any color), tops cut off and seeds removed
- 1 cup cooked brown rice
- 1 small onion, finely chopped
- 2 garlic cloves, minced
- 1 medium tomato, diced
- 2 tbsp chopped fresh parsley
- 1 tbsp chopped fresh mint
- 2 tbsp olive oil
- 1 tsp dried oregano
- Salt and black pepper, to taste
- ½ cup crumbled feta cheese
- ½ cup vegetable broth or water (for baking)

Directions

- Preheat your oven to 375°F (190°C).
- In a large skillet, heat 1 tablespoon of olive oil over medium heat. Add chopped onion and garlic. Sauté for 3–4 minutes until softened.
- Stir in the cooked rice, diced tomato, parsley, mint (if using), oregano, salt, and pepper. Cook for another 2–3 minutes until everything is well combined and warmed through.
- Remove from heat and mix in the feta cheese, if using.
- Fill each bell pepper with the rice mixture and place them upright in a baking dish.
- Drizzle the remaining 1 tablespoon of olive oil over the peppers and pour the vegetable broth or water into the bottom of the dish.
- Cover the dish with foil and bake for 30–35 minutes until the peppers are tender.
- Remove the foil during the last 5–10 minutes to lightly brown the tops.

Tips

- For a protein boost, add cooked lentils or ground turkey to the filling.
- Use leftover rice or quinoa to save time.
- These stuffed peppers can be made ahead and reheated – they taste even better the next day!
- Swap feta for goat cheese or omit for a dairy-free version.

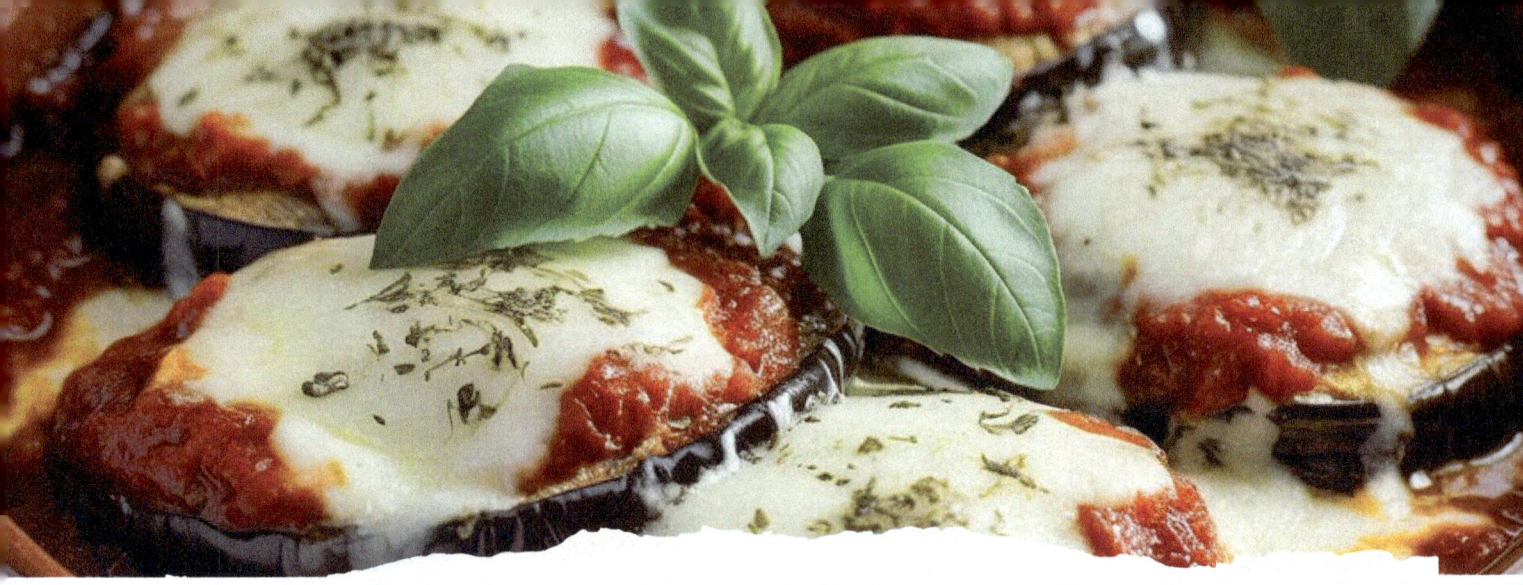

EGGPLANT PARMESAN (BAKED, NOT FRIED)

Servings: 4 **Total Time:** 1 Hour

Calories: 310 | **Protein:** 16g | **Carbohydrates:** 25g | **Fat:** 17g

Ingredients

- 2 medium eggplants, sliced into ½-inch rounds
- 1 teaspoon salt
- 1½ cups marinara sauce (low-sodium if possible)
- 1½ cups shredded mozzarella cheese
- ½ cup grated Parmesan cheese
- 1 cup whole wheat breadcrumbs
- 2 eggs, beaten
- 1 tablespoon extra virgin olive oil
- 1 teaspoon dried oregano
- ½ teaspoon garlic powder
- Fresh basil leaves for garnish

Tips

- Use a low-sodium marinara to control salt levels, especially important for seniors.
- For extra crispiness, toast breadcrumbs in a dry pan before coating.
- Want to make it gluten-free? Use gluten-free breadcrumbs.
- Make it ahead! Assemble the dish and refrigerate, then bake when ready to serve.

Directions

- **Prepare Eggplant:** Sprinkle eggplant slices with salt and place in a colander. Let sit for 20 minutes to draw out moisture. Pat dry with paper towels.
- **Preheat Oven:** Set oven to 400°F (200°C). Line a baking sheet with parchment paper and lightly brush with olive oil.
- **Coat Slices:** Dip eggplant slices into beaten eggs, then coat with breadcrumbs mixed with oregano and garlic powder.
- **Bake:** Arrange slices on the prepared baking sheet. Bake for 20 minutes, flipping halfway through until golden and tender.
- **Assemble:** In a baking dish, spread a thin layer of marinara. Add a layer of baked eggplant, then spoon marinara on top, sprinkle mozzarella and Parmesan. Repeat layers.
- **Bake Again:** Cover loosely with foil and bake for 15 minutes. Remove foil and bake an additional 10 minutes, or until cheese is bubbly and slightly golden.
- **Serve:** Let rest for 5 minutes. Garnish with fresh basil if desired and serve warm.

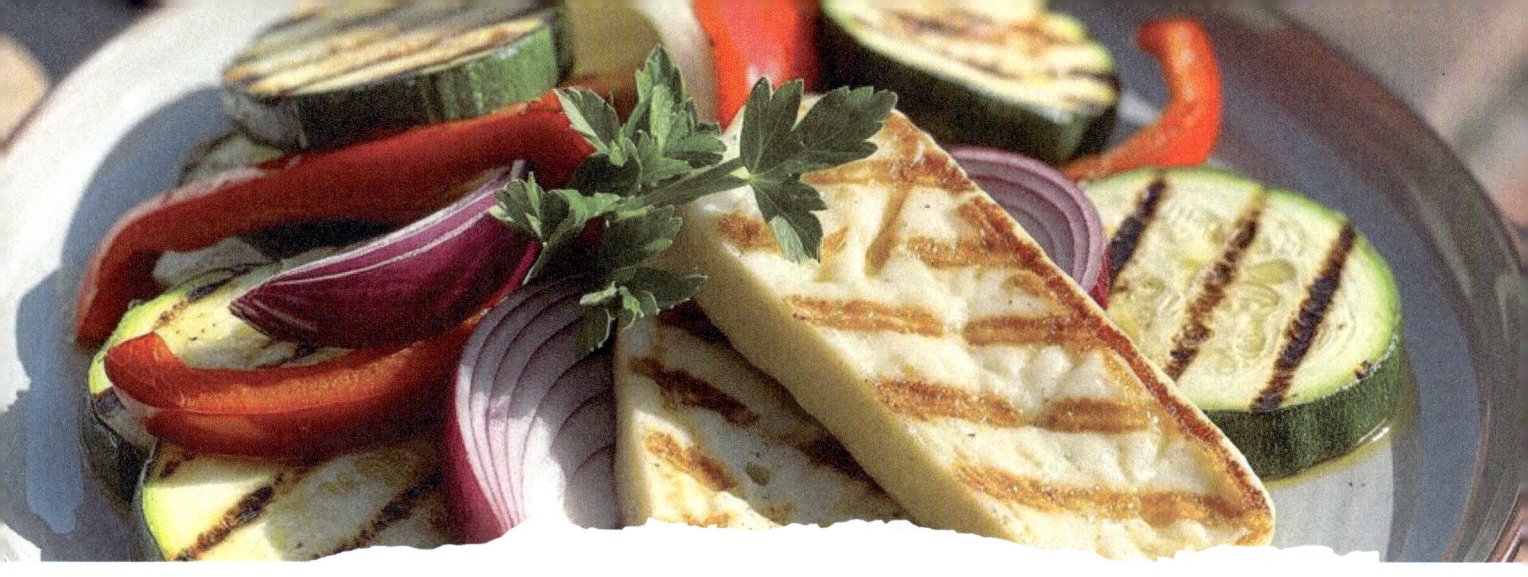

GRILLED HALLOUMI WITH VEGETABLES

Servings: 2 **Total Time:** 25 Min

Calories: 320 | **Protein:** 16g | **Carbohydrates:** 12g | **Fat:** 24g

Ingredients

- 200g halloumi cheese, sliced into ½-inch thick pieces
- 1 medium zucchini, sliced into rounds
- 1 red bell pepper, sliced into strips
- 1 small red onion, cut into wedges
- 1 tbsp olive oil
- ½ tsp dried oregano
- Juice of ½ lemon
- Salt and black pepper to taste
- Fresh parsley for garnish

Directions

- Preheat the grill or a grill pan over medium heat.
- In a bowl, toss the zucchini, bell pepper, and onion with olive oil, oregano, salt, and pepper.
- Place the vegetables on the grill and cook for 4–5 minutes per side, or until tender and lightly charred. Remove and set aside.
- Grill the halloumi slices for 2–3 minutes on each side until golden brown and slightly crispy on the outside.
- Arrange the grilled vegetables and halloumi on a serving plate. Drizzle with lemon juice and garnish with fresh parsley if desired.
- Serve warm as a main or a side dish.

Tips

- Use a grill basket or foil to prevent small veggie pieces from falling through the grill.
- Add cherry tomatoes or mushrooms for extra variety.
- For a heartier meal, serve with a side of quinoa or whole grain couscous.
- Halloumi grills best when it's dry – pat it with a paper towel before grilling.

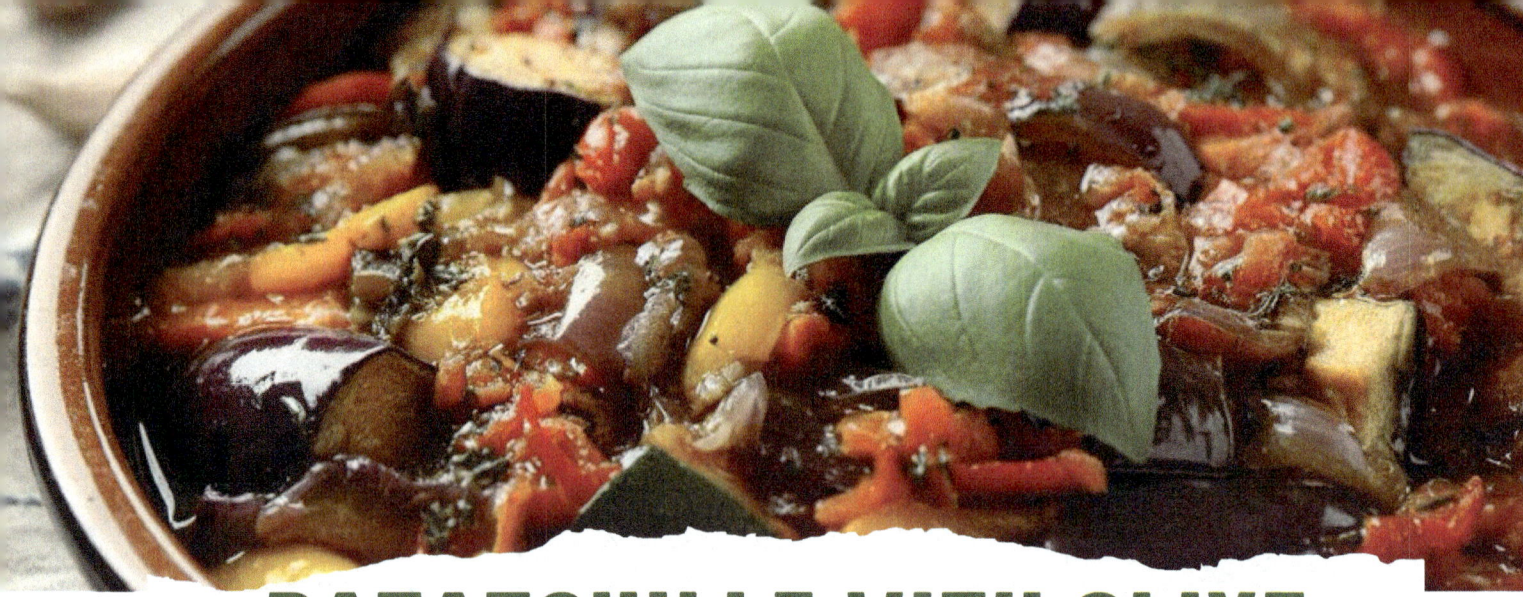

RATATOUILLE WITH OLIVE OIL AND BASIL

Servings: 4 | **Total Time:** 45 Min

Calories: 130 | **Protein:** 3g | **Carbohydrates:** 15g | **Fat:** 8g

Ingredients

- 1 medium eggplant, diced
- 1 zucchini, sliced
- 1 yellow squash, sliced
- 1 red bell pepper, chopped
- 1 green bell pepper, chopped
- 1 medium onion, sliced
- 3 garlic cloves, minced
- 2 tablespoons extra-virgin olive oil
- 1 (14.5 oz) can diced tomatoes (or 3 fresh tomatoes, chopped)
- 1 teaspoon dried oregano
- Salt and pepper to taste
- Fresh basil leaves, chopped (for garnish)

Directions

- Heat olive oil in a large skillet over medium heat.
- Add onions and garlic; sauté for 2–3 minutes until fragrant.
- Add eggplant and cook for 5–7 minutes until it begins to soften.
- Add zucchini, yellow squash, and bell peppers. Cook for another 7–10 minutes, stirring occasionally.
- Stir in diced tomatoes and oregano. Season with salt and pepper.
- Cover and simmer for 15 minutes, until vegetables are tender and the flavors are well combined.
- Remove from heat, sprinkle with fresh basil, and serve warm.

Tips

- For added richness, roast the vegetables beforehand and then simmer together.
- Serve with a slice of whole grain bread or over brown rice for a complete meal.
- Leftovers taste even better the next day as the flavors continue to develop.

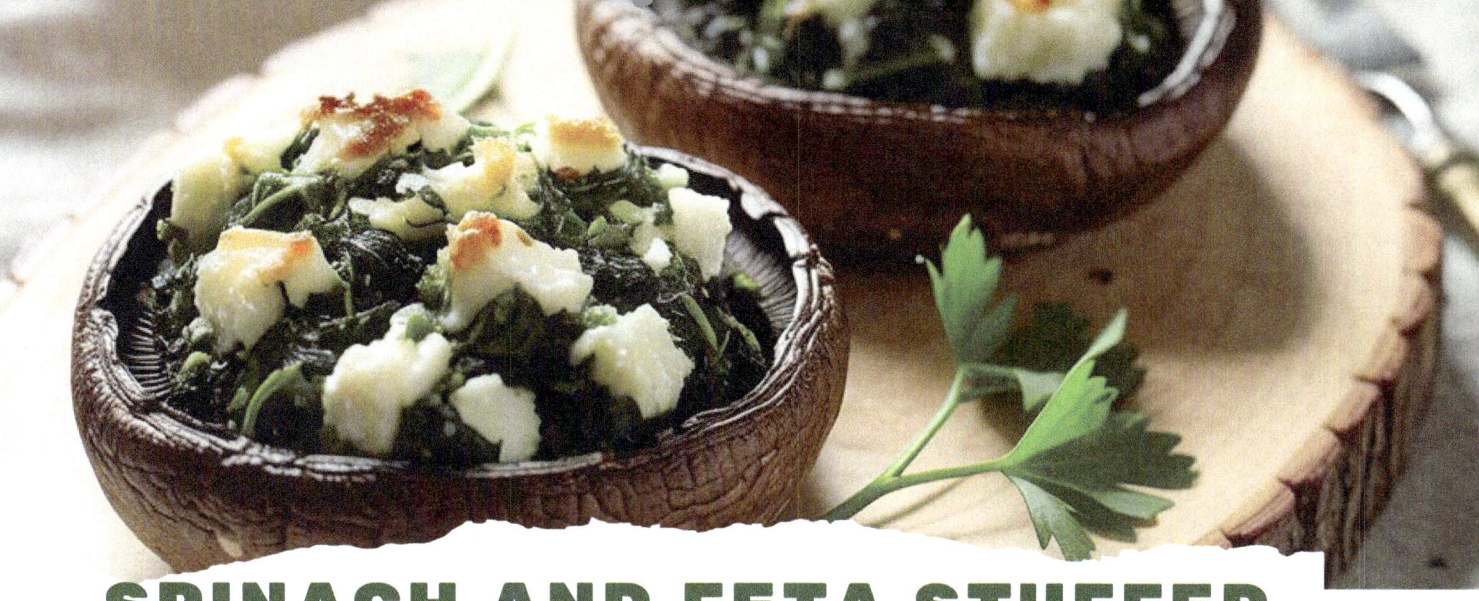

SPINACH AND FETA STUFFED PORTOBELLOS

Servings: 2 | **Total Time:** 30 Min

Calories: ~180 | **Protein:** 8g | **Carbohydrates:** 7g | **Fat:** 13g

Ingredients

- 2 large Portobello mushroom caps, stems removed and gills scraped out
- 1 tablespoon olive oil
- 2 cups fresh spinach, chopped
- 1 garlic clove, minced
- 1/4 cup crumbled feta cheese
- 2 tablespoons grated Parmesan cheese (optional)
- 1 tablespoon chopped fresh parsley (or 1 tsp dried)
- Salt and black pepper to taste
- Olive oil spray (optional, for baking)

Tips

- For a protein boost, add cooked quinoa or shredded chicken to the filling.
- These make a great meatless main dish or a hearty side.
- Use baby spinach for quicker cooking and easier texture.
- You can prep the filling ahead and refrigerate for up to 1 day before stuffing the mushrooms.

Directions

- Preheat your oven to 375°F (190°C).
- Brush the Portobello caps with olive oil on both sides and place them on a baking sheet, gill side up.
- In a skillet over medium heat, sauté garlic in a little olive oil for 30 seconds, then add the chopped spinach. Cook until wilted, about 2–3 minutes.
- Remove from heat and stir in the crumbled feta, Parmesan (if using), and chopped parsley. Season with salt and pepper.
- Spoon the spinach-feta mixture evenly into each mushroom cap.
- Lightly spray the tops with olive oil and bake for 15–20 minutes, or until the mushrooms are tender and the filling is golden.
- Serve warm, garnished with a few extra parsley leaves if desired.

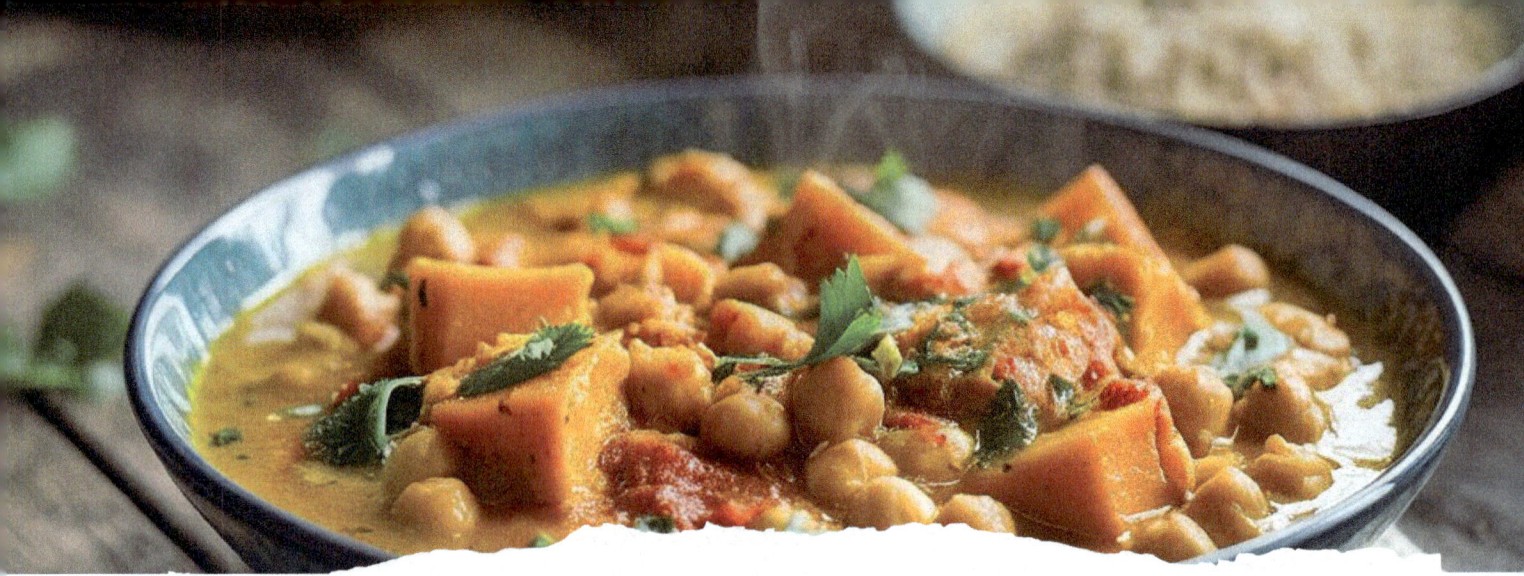

CHICKPEA AND SWEET POTATO CURRY

Servings: 4   **Total Time:** 35 Min

Calories: 320 | **Protein:** 9g | **Carbohydrates:** 45g | **Fat:** 12g

Ingredients

- 1 tablespoon olive oil
- 1 small onion, finely chopped
- 2 cloves garlic, minced
- 1 tablespoon grated fresh ginger
- 2 teaspoons curry powder
- 1 teaspoon ground cumin
- 1/2 teaspoon paprika
- 1 large sweet potato, peeled and diced
- 1 can (15 oz) chickpeas, drained and rinsed
- 1 can (14 oz) diced tomatoes
- 1/2 cup low-sodium vegetable broth or water
- 1/2 cup light coconut milk
- Salt and pepper to taste
- Fresh cilantro or parsley, chopped
- Cooked brown rice or quinoa, for serving

Directions

- Heat olive oil in a large skillet over medium heat. Add chopped onion and sauté for 3–4 minutes until softened.
- Stir in garlic and ginger, cooking for another 1 minute until fragrant.
- Add curry powder, cumin, and paprika. Stir well to coat the onions in the spices.
- Add the diced sweet potatoes, chickpeas, diced tomatoes (with juice), broth, and coconut milk. Stir to combine.
- Bring to a gentle boil, then reduce heat, cover, and simmer for 20–25 minutes or until the sweet potatoes are tender.
- Season with salt and pepper to taste.
- Serve hot, garnished with fresh herbs if desired, over brown rice or quinoa.

Tips

- For a protein boost, add cooked quinoa or shredded chicken to the filling.
- These make a great meatless main dish or a hearty side.
- Use baby spinach for quicker cooking and easier texture.
- You can prep the filling ahead and refrigerate for up to 1 day before stuffing the mushrooms.

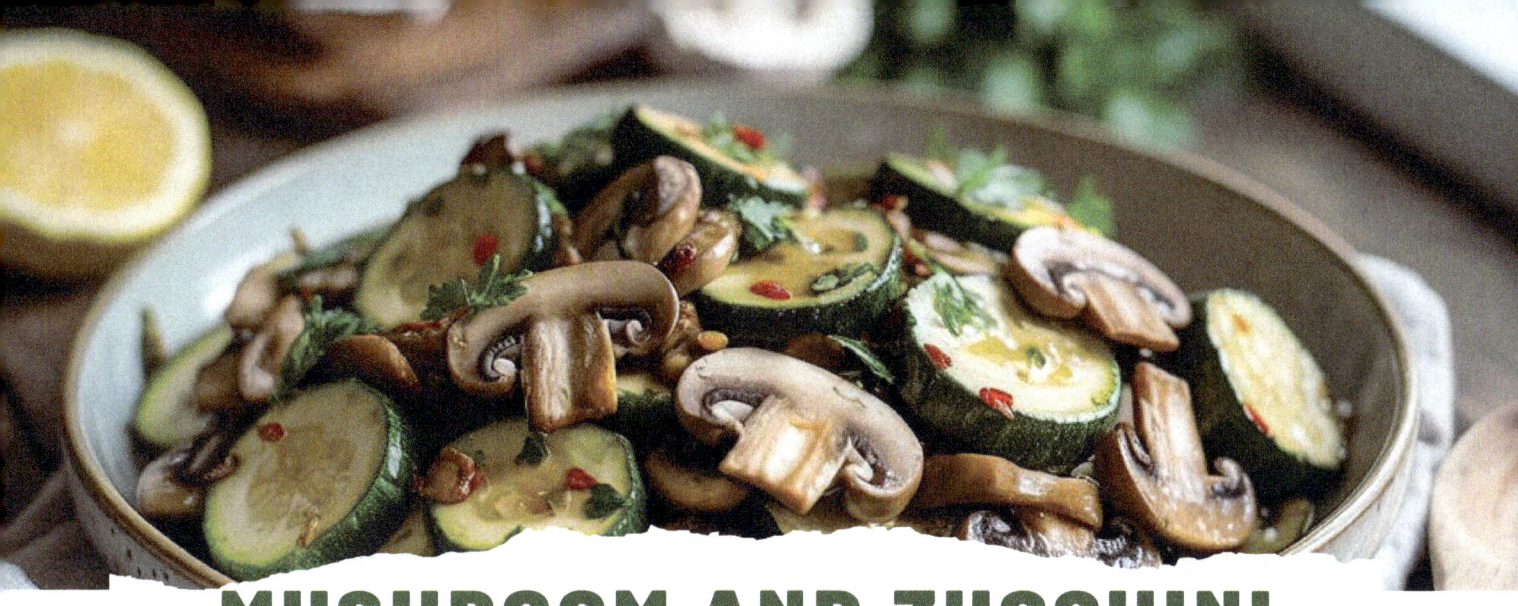

MUSHROOM AND ZUCCHINI STIR-FRY

Servings: 2   **Total Time:** 20 Min

Calories: 110 | **Protein:** 3g | **Carbohydrates:** 8g | **Fat:** 7g

Ingredients

- 1 tablespoon extra-virgin olive oil
- 2 cups sliced mushrooms (button or cremini)
- 1 medium zucchini, sliced into thin rounds
- 2 cloves garlic, minced
- 1 teaspoon dried oregano
- Salt and pepper to taste
- 1 tablespoon chopped fresh parsley
- A squeeze of fresh lemon juice

Directions

- Heat the olive oil in a large skillet over medium heat.
- Add the garlic and sauté for 30 seconds until fragrant.
- Add the sliced mushrooms and cook for 5–6 minutes, stirring occasionally, until they release their moisture and begin to brown.
- Add the zucchini slices and oregano. Continue to cook for another 5–7 minutes until the zucchini is tender but not mushy.
- Season with salt and pepper to taste.
- Remove from heat and garnish with fresh parsley and a squeeze of lemon juice if desired.
- Serve warm as a light main or a hearty side.

Tips

- Add a handful of baby spinach in the last minute of cooking for extra greens.
- Pair this with whole grain couscous or quinoa for a more filling meal.
- Use a nonstick skillet to reduce the amount of oil needed.

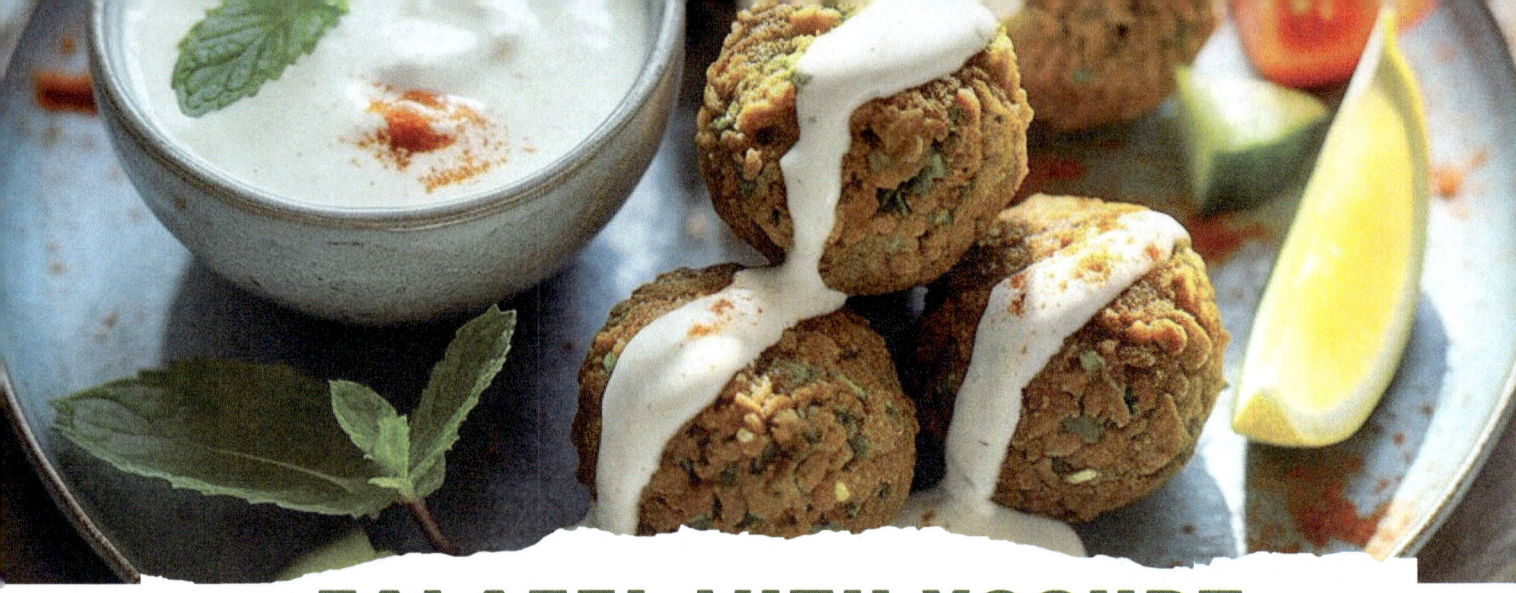

FALAFEL WITH YOGURT SAUCE

Servings: 4 | **Total Time:** 45 Min

Calories: 290 | **Protein:** 12g | **Carbohydrates:** 30g | **Fat:** 14g

Ingredients

For the Falafel:
- 1 cup dried chickpeas (soaked overnight and drained)
- 1 small onion, chopped
- 3 cloves garlic, minced
- 1/2 cup fresh parsley
- 1/2 cup fresh cilantro
- 1 tsp ground cumin
- 1 tsp ground coriander
- 1/2 tsp baking powder
- Salt and pepper, to taste
- 2–3 tbsp olive oil (for frying or baking)

For the Yogurt Sauce:
- 1 cup plain Greek yogurt
- 1 tbsp lemon juice
- 1 small garlic clove, minced
- 1 tbsp chopped fresh mint or dill
- Salt, to taste

Directions

- **Make the falafel mixture:** In a food processor, combine soaked chickpeas, onion, garlic, parsley, cilantro, cumin, coriander, salt, and pepper. Pulse until the mixture forms a coarse paste.
- **Add baking powder:** Transfer mixture to a bowl. Stir in baking powder. Chill in the fridge for 15–20 minutes.
- **Form falafel balls:** Use a spoon or your hands to shape into small balls or patties.
- **Cook:** *To pan-fry:* Heat olive oil in a skillet over medium heat. Fry falafel for 3–4 minutes per side until golden brown.
- **To bake:** Preheat oven to 375°F (190°C). Place falafel on a lined baking sheet, brush with olive oil, and bake for 25–30 minutes, flipping halfway.
- **Make the yogurt sauce:** In a small bowl, combine yogurt, lemon juice, garlic, herbs, and salt. Mix well.
- **Serve:** Serve falafel warm with the yogurt sauce on the side or drizzled on top.

Tips

- Don't use canned chickpeas – they're too soft. Dried and soaked chickpeas give the best texture.
- You can freeze uncooked falafel balls for up to 1 month.
- Serve with pita bread, lettuce, cucumber, and tomato for a complete meal.

BAKED FETA WITH CHERRY TOMATOES

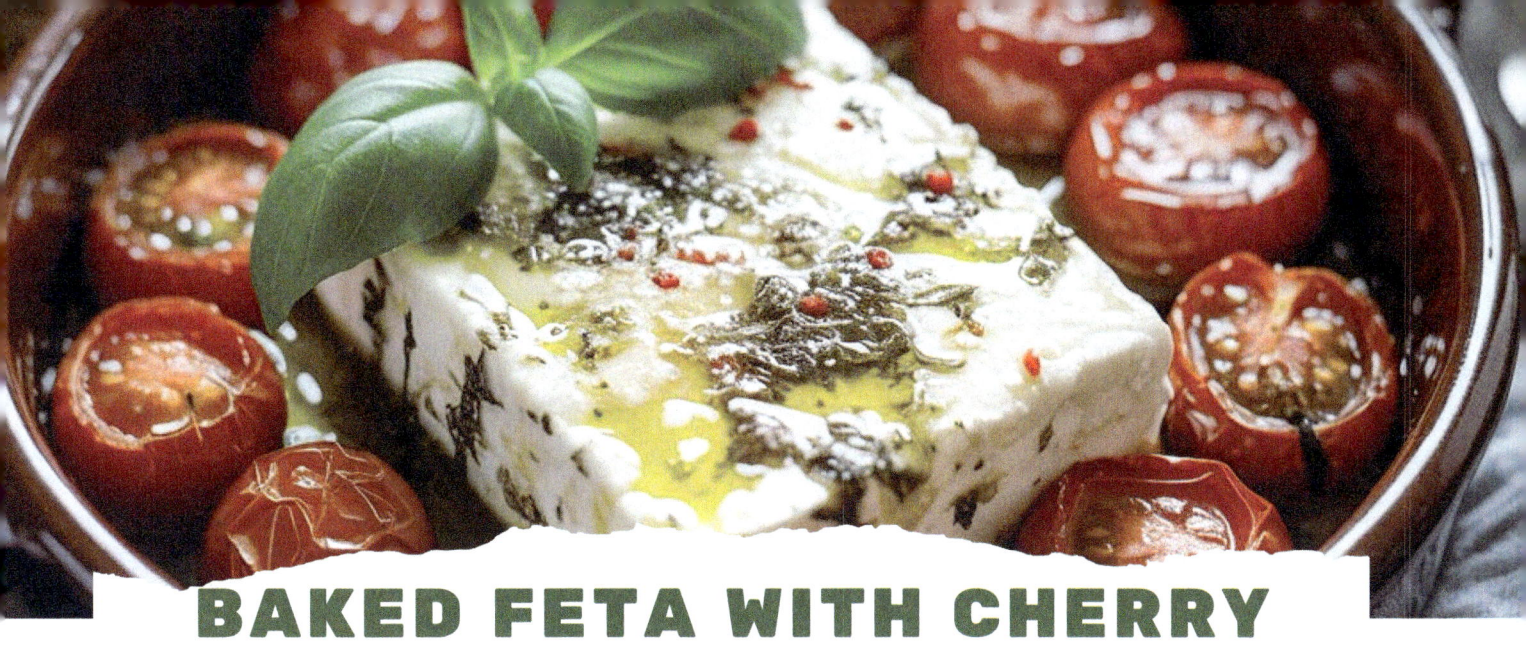

Servings: 2   **Total Time:** 30 Min

Calories: 280 | **Protein:** 9g | **Fat:** 24g | **Carbohydrates:** 8g

Ingredients

- 1 block (7 oz) feta cheese
- 2 cups cherry tomatoes, whole or halved
- 3 tablespoons extra-virgin olive oil
- 2 garlic cloves, minced
- 1 teaspoon dried oregano
- ¼ teaspoon crushed red pepper flakes
- Freshly ground black pepper, to taste
- Fresh basil leaves, for garnish
- Whole grain bread or pita, for serving

Directions

- Preheat your oven to 400°F (200°C).
- In a small baking dish, place the block of feta in the center.
- Surround the feta with cherry tomatoes, then drizzle olive oil evenly over the cheese and tomatoes.
- Sprinkle the garlic, oregano, crushed red pepper flakes (if using), and black pepper on top.
- Bake for 25 minutes, or until the tomatoes are blistered and the feta is soft and golden on top.
- Remove from oven, gently mix the melted feta and tomatoes together if desired.
- Garnish with fresh basil leaves and serve warm with whole grain bread or pita.

Tips

- For added flavor, toss in a few olives before baking.
- Use a good quality block of feta – avoid crumbled feta for this recipe.
- This dish also pairs beautifully with cooked pasta or quinoa for a more filling meal.
- Leftovers can be refrigerated and enjoyed cold or reheated the next day.

LENTIL AND VEGGIE PATTIES

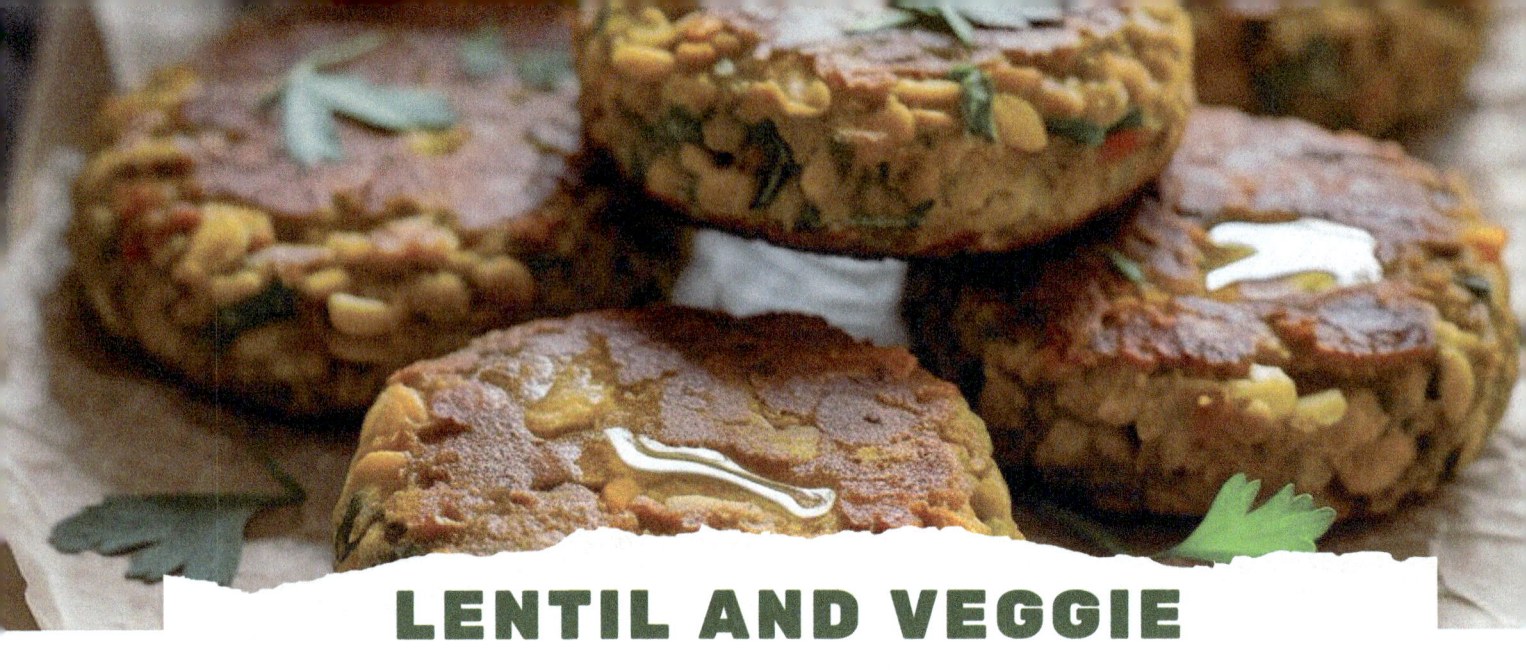

Servings: 4   **Total Time:** 35 Min

Calories: 210 | **Protein:** 10g | **Carbohydrates:** 22g | **Fat:** 10g

Ingredients

- 1 cup cooked lentils (green or brown)
- 1 small carrot, grated
- 1 small zucchini, grated and squeezed dry
- 1/4 cup chopped red onion
- 1 garlic clove, minced
- 1/4 cup breadcrumbs (whole wheat preferred)
- 1 egg
- 1 tablespoon chopped fresh parsley
- 1/2 teaspoon cumin
- Salt and pepper, to taste
- 2 tablespoons olive oil (for cooking)

Directions

- In a large bowl, mash the cooked lentils with a fork until chunky but not completely smooth.
- Add grated carrot, zucchini, red onion, garlic, breadcrumbs, egg, parsley, cumin, salt, and pepper. Mix well until combined.
- Form the mixture into 6–8 small patties using your hands.
- Heat olive oil in a non-stick skillet over medium heat.
- Cook the patties for 4–5 minutes on each side, or until golden brown and cooked through.
- Remove from skillet and place on paper towels to drain excess oil. Serve warm.

Tips

- You can use canned lentils for a quicker prep—just rinse and drain them well.
- Want to make it vegan? Replace the egg with a flax egg (1 tbsp ground flax + 2.5 tbsp water).
- Serve with Greek yogurt or a simple tahini sauce for added flavor.
- These patties freeze well! Let them cool, then freeze in a single layer for up to 2 months.

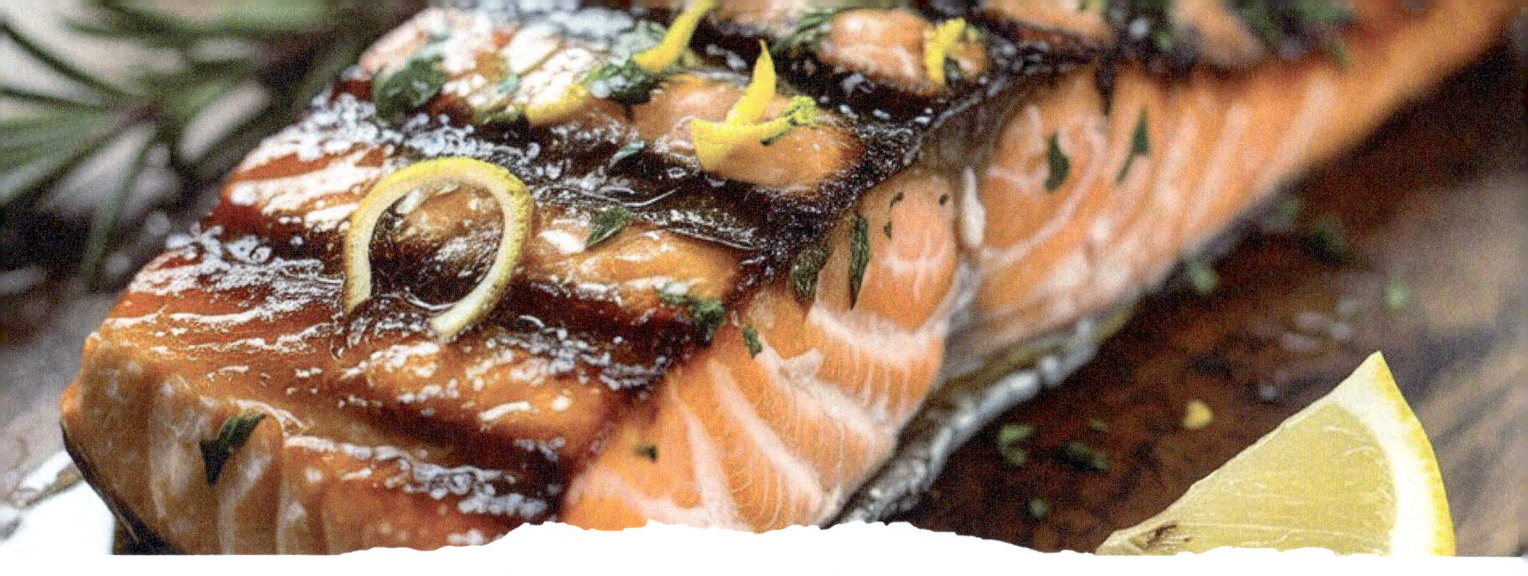

GRILLED LEMON HERB SALMON

Servings: 2   **Total Time:** 25 Min

Calories: 320 | **Protein:** 34g | **Fat:** 18g | **Carbohydrates:** 2g

Ingredients

- 2 salmon fillets (about 5–6 oz each)
- 2 tablespoons extra-virgin olive oil
- Juice of 1 lemon
- 1 teaspoon lemon zest
- 2 garlic cloves, minced
- 1 tablespoon fresh parsley, chopped
- 1 teaspoon dried oregano
- Salt and pepper, to taste
- Lemon slices, for garnish

Tips

- For extra flavor, add a few fresh dill sprigs to the marinade.
- If you don't have a grill, this recipe works well in a skillet or baked in the oven at 400°F (200°C) for 12–15 minutes.
- Always use fresh lemon juice for the best taste.

Directions

- **Prepare the marinade:** In a small bowl, whisk together olive oil, lemon juice, lemon zest, garlic, parsley, oregano, salt, and pepper.
- **Marinate the salmon:** Place salmon fillets in a shallow dish or zip-lock bag. Pour the marinade over the fillets and let them sit for 15–20 minutes (do not over-marinate).
- **Preheat the grill:** ·Heat your grill or grill pan over medium heat. Lightly oil the grates.
- **Grill the salmon:** Remove the fillets from the marinade and place them skin-side down on the grill. Grill for about 4–5 minutes per side, or until the salmon flakes easily with a fork.
- **Serve:** Transfer to plates and garnish with fresh lemon slices if desired. Serve with a side of veggies or whole grains.

BAKED COD WITH TOMATOES AND OLIVES

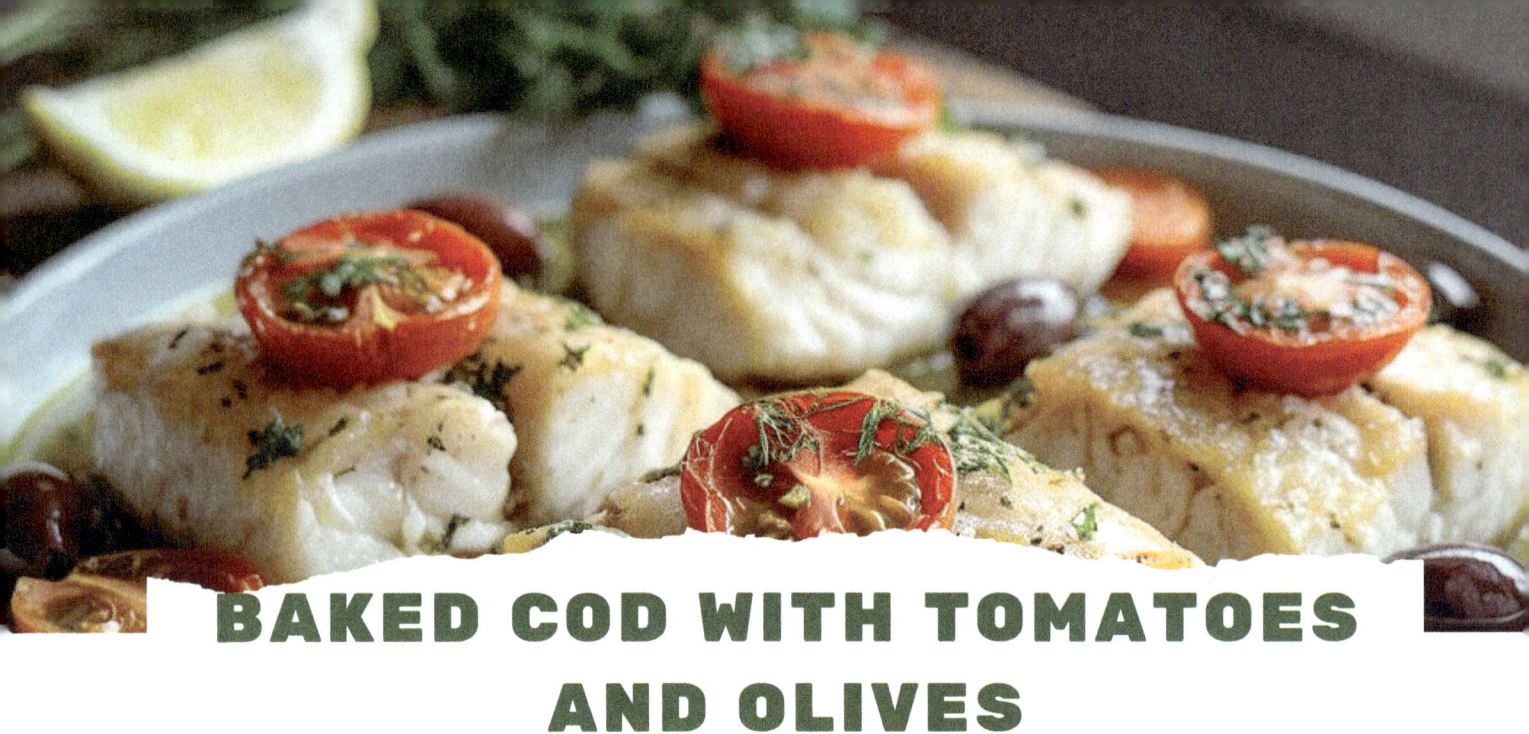

Servings: 4 | **Total Time:** 30 Min

Calories: 260 | **Protein:** 30g | **Fat:** 12g | **Carbohydrates:** 6g

Ingredients

- 4 cod fillets (about 5–6 oz each)
- 2 cups cherry tomatoes, halved
- 1/2 cup Kalamata olives, pitted and sliced
- 3 garlic cloves, minced
- 2 tablespoons extra-virgin olive oil
- 1 tablespoon fresh lemon juice
- 1 teaspoon dried oregano
- Salt and black pepper to taste
- Fresh parsley, chopped (for garnish)

Directions

- Preheat oven to 400°F (200°C).
- Place the cod fillets in a baking dish and season both sides with salt and pepper.
- In a bowl, combine cherry tomatoes, olives, garlic, olive oil, lemon juice, and oregano.
- Spoon the tomato-olive mixture over the fish evenly.
- Bake for 18–20 minutes, or until the cod is opaque and flakes easily with a fork.
- Garnish with fresh parsley before serving. Serve warm with a side of steamed vegetables or whole grains.

Tips

- Swap cod for haddock or halibut if preferred.
- Add a handful of baby spinach to the baking dish for extra greens.
- For a spicier version, sprinkle with crushed red pepper flakes before baking.

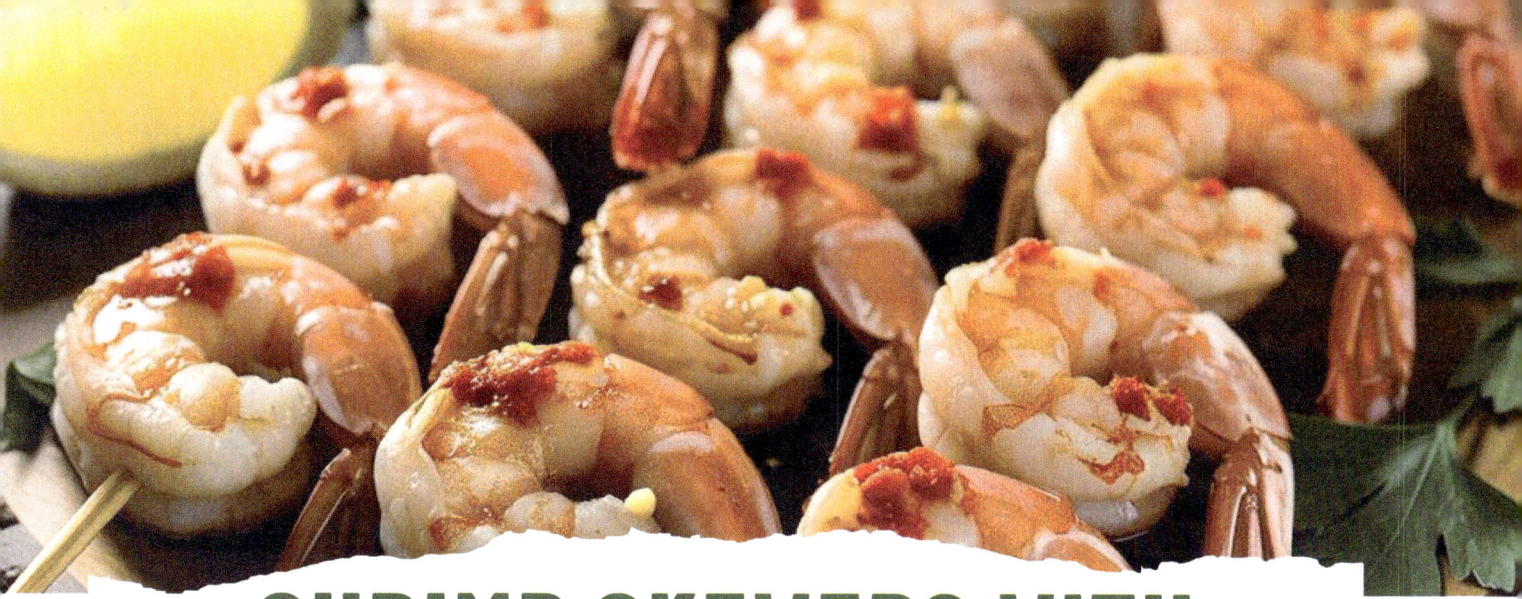

SHRIMP SKEWERS WITH GARLIC AND PAPRIKA

Servings: 4   **Total Time:** 25 Min

Calories: 180 | **Protein:** 22g | **Carbohydrates:** 2g | **Fat:** 9g

Ingredients

- 1 lb (450g) large shrimp, peeled and deveined
- 2 tablespoons olive oil
- 3 cloves garlic, minced
- 1 teaspoon smoked paprika
- ½ teaspoon ground cumin
- Juice of ½ lemon
- Salt and black pepper, to taste
- Fresh parsley, chopped (for garnish)
- Lemon wedges, for serving
- Wooden or metal skewers (if using wooden, soak in water for 30 minutes)

Directions

- **Prepare the marinade:** In a large bowl, combine olive oil, garlic, paprika, cumin, lemon juice, salt, and pepper.
- **Marinate the shrimp:** Add the shrimp to the bowl and toss to coat evenly. Let sit for 10–15 minutes while you heat the grill or grill pan.
- **Assemble the skewers:** Thread the marinated shrimp onto skewers, leaving a little space between each one.
- **Grill the shrimp:** Heat a grill or grill pan over medium-high heat. Grill the skewers for 2–3 minutes per side, or until the shrimp are pink and cooked through.
- **Garnish and serve:** Remove from heat, sprinkle with fresh parsley, and serve with lemon wedges.

Tips

- For extra flavor, marinate the shrimp for up to 1 hour in the refrigerator.
- Add colorful veggies like bell peppers or zucchini between shrimp on skewers.
- Serve with a side of quinoa, couscous, or a fresh Mediterranean salad for a complete meal.

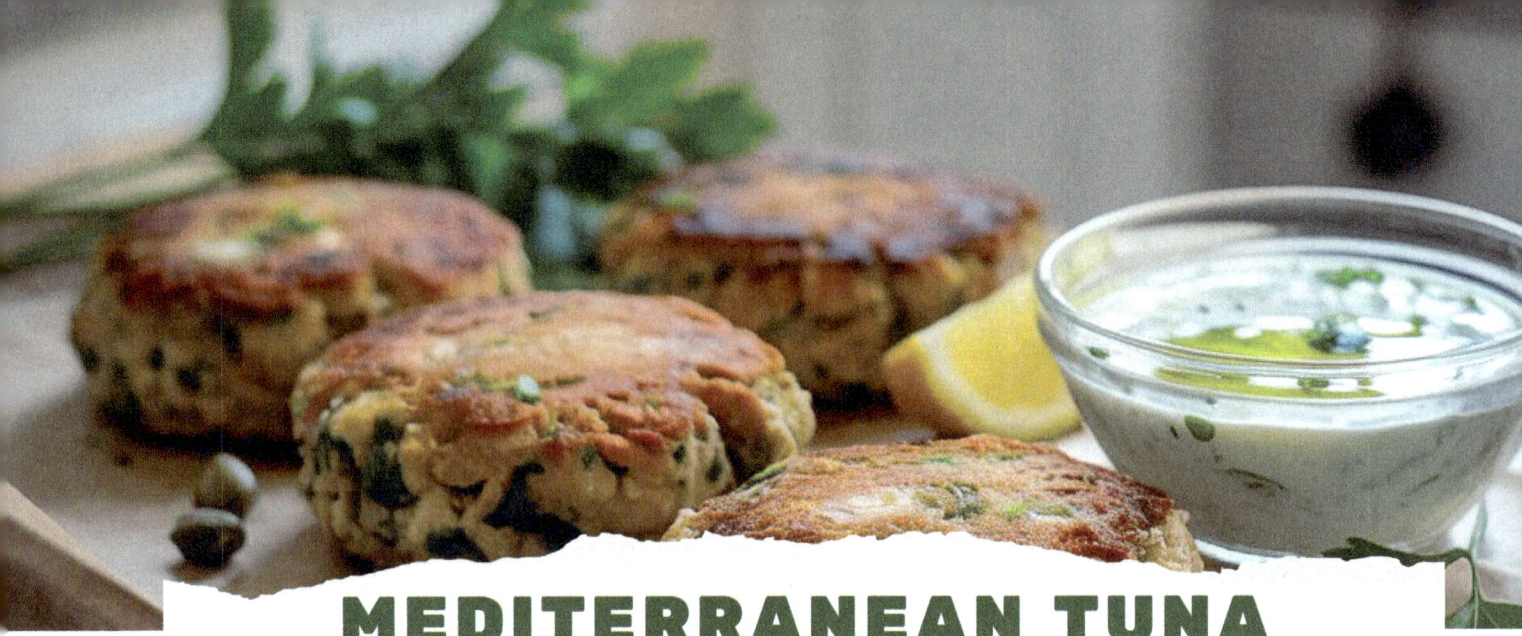

MEDITERRANEAN TUNA PATTIES

Servings: 4   **Total Time:** 25 Min

Calories: 230 | **Protein:** 25g | **Fat:** 10g | **Carbohydrates:** 8g

Ingredients

- 2 cans (5 oz each) tuna in water, drained
- 1/4 cup breadcrumbs (whole wheat if preferred)
- 1 large egg
- 1/4 cup red onion, finely chopped
- 2 tablespoons parsley, chopped
- 1 tablespoon capers, chopped (optional)
- 1 teaspoon Dijon mustard
- 1 teaspoon lemon juice
- 1/2 teaspoon garlic powder
- Salt and pepper to taste
- 1 tablespoon olive oil (for cooking)

Directions

- In a medium bowl, combine drained tuna, breadcrumbs, egg, red onion, parsley, capers (if using), mustard, lemon juice, garlic powder, salt, and pepper.
- Mix well with a fork or clean hands until the mixture holds together.
- Shape the mixture into 4 small patties.
- Heat olive oil in a skillet over medium heat.
- Cook the patties for about 3–4 minutes per side or until golden brown and cooked through.
- Serve warm with a side salad, whole grain pita, or yogurt sauce.

Tips

- Add chopped sun-dried tomatoes or olives for extra flavor.
- For a gluten-free version, use almond flour or gluten-free breadcrumbs.
- These patties store well in the fridge and can be reheated for up to 3 days.
- Serve with tzatziki or a lemon-garlic yogurt sauce for a refreshing twist.

SARDINES WITH LEMON AND PARSLEY

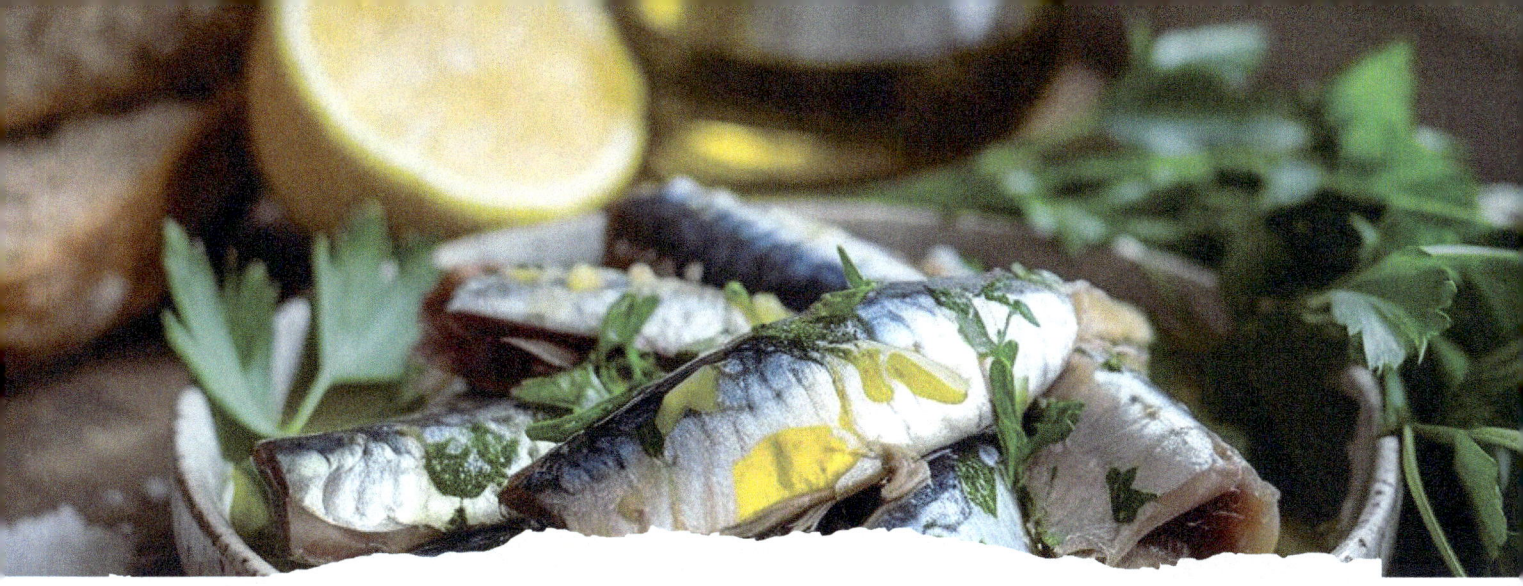

Servings: 2   **Total Time:** 15 Min

Calories: 180 | **Protein:** 18g | **Fat:** 12g | **Carbohydrates:** 1g

Ingredients

- 1 can (4 oz) sardines in olive oil (drained)
- 1 tablespoon fresh lemon juice
- 1 teaspoon lemon zest
- 1 tablespoon fresh parsley, finely chopped
- 1 clove garlic, minced (optional)
- 1 tablespoon extra-virgin olive oil
- Salt and black pepper to taste
- Whole grain bread or crackers for serving

Directions

- In a small bowl, gently mix the drained sardines with lemon juice, lemon zest, parsley, and garlic (if using).
- Drizzle the olive oil over the mixture and season lightly with salt and black pepper.
- Let it sit for 5 minutes to allow the flavors to meld.
- Serve on its own, or over warm whole grain bread or crackers for a quick and satisfying Mediterranean snack or light lunch.

Tips

- Use fresh sardines if available and grill them briefly for added flavor.
- Add a pinch of chili flakes if you like a touch of heat.
- For a heartier meal, serve over a bed of quinoa or a simple green salad.

FISH TACOS WITH YOGURT DILL SAUCE

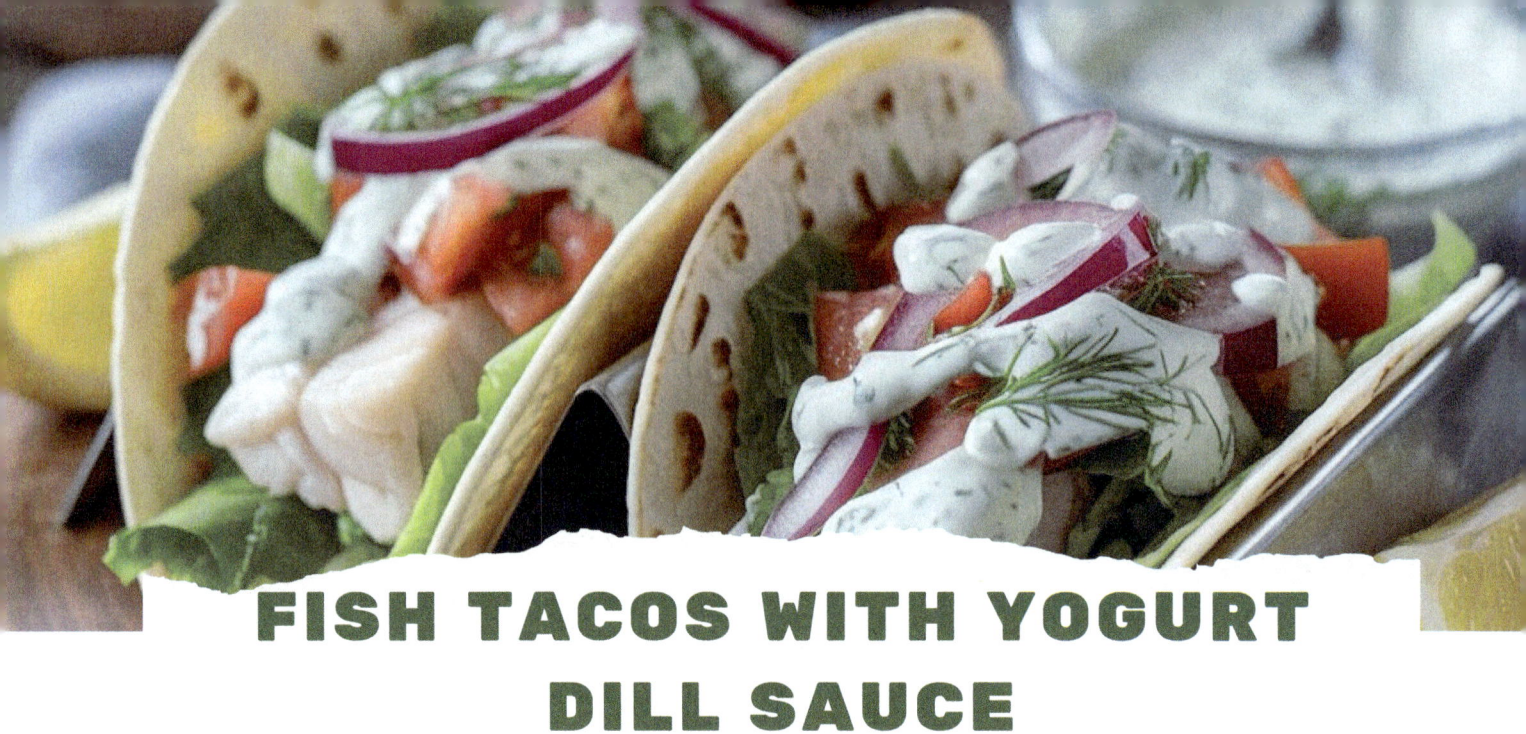

Servings: 2 **Total Time:** 25 Min

Calories: 350 | **Protein:** 28g | **Carbohydrates:** 25g | **Fat:** 15g

Ingredients

For the Fish:
- 2 white fish fillets (such as cod or tilapia)
- 1 tablespoon olive oil
- 1 teaspoon paprika
- ½ teaspoon garlic powder
- Salt and black pepper, to taste
- Juice of ½ lemon

For the Yogurt Dill Sauce:
- ½ cup plain Greek yogurt
- 1 tablespoon fresh dill (or 1 teaspoon dried)
- 1 teaspoon lemon juice
- 1 small garlic clove, minced
- Salt to taste

For Assembly:
- 4 small whole wheat tortillas
- ½ cup shredded lettuce or cabbage
- ½ cup diced tomatoes
- ¼ cup sliced red onion
- Optional: avocado slices or feta cheese

Directions

- **Prepare the Fish:** Pat fish fillets dry. Rub with olive oil, paprika, garlic powder, salt, pepper, and lemon juice.
- Heat a nonstick skillet over medium heat and cook the fillets for 3–4 minutes per side or until cooked through and flaky. Remove from pan and set aside.
- **Make the Sauce:** In a small bowl, mix Greek yogurt, dill, lemon juice, garlic, and a pinch of salt. Stir until creamy and well combined.
- **Assemble Tacos:** Warm tortillas in a pan or microwave.
- Flake the cooked fish into chunks and divide evenly among the tortillas.
- Top with lettuce, tomatoes, onions, and a generous spoon of the yogurt dill sauce. Add avocado or feta if desired.
- **Serve:** Serve warm with a lemon wedge on the side.

Tips

- For extra crunch, use red cabbage instead of lettuce.
- You can grill the fish for added smokiness.
- Add a pinch of cayenne pepper to the yogurt sauce for a spicy kick.
- This dish works great with leftover fish or even canned tuna in a pinch.

MUSSELS IN TOMATO WINE BROTH

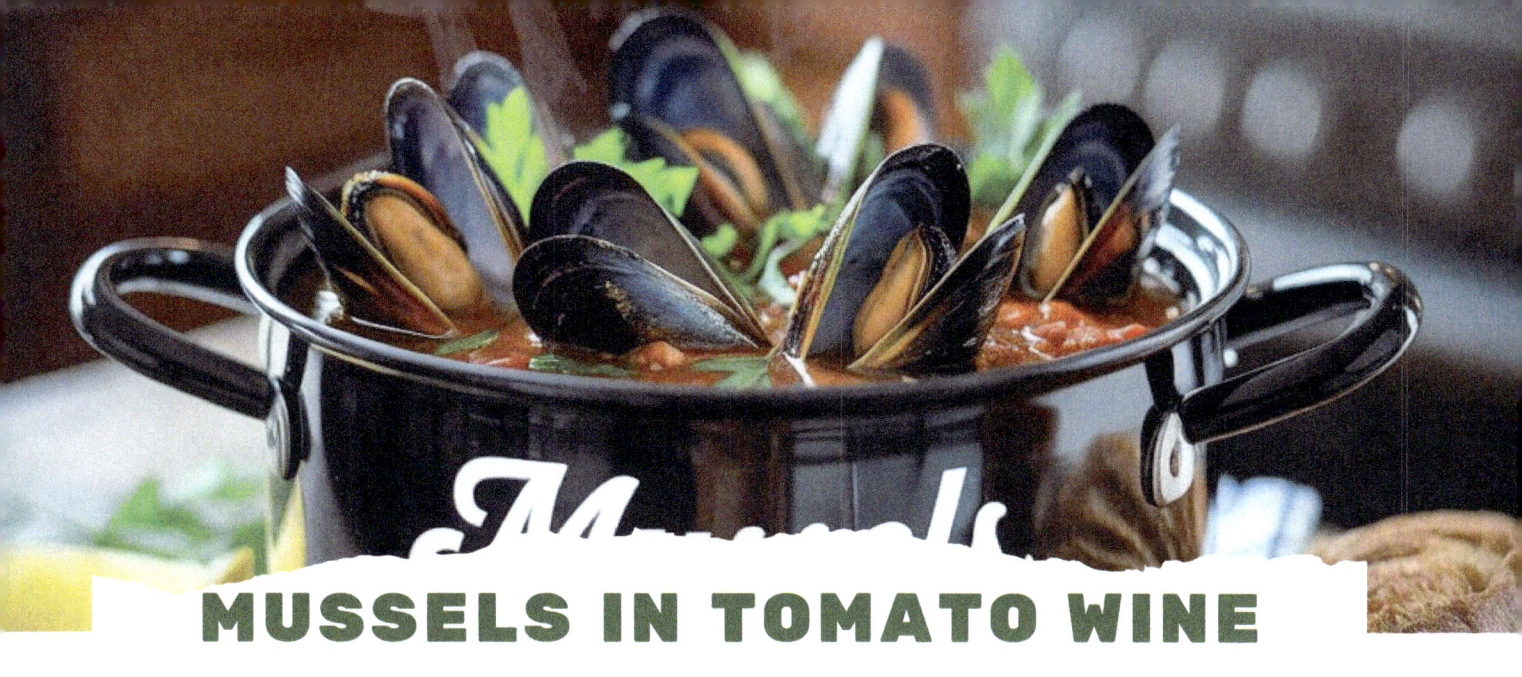

Servings: 2 **Total Time:** 25 Min

Calories: 290 | **Protein:** 22g | **Carbohydrates:** 12g | **Fat:** 15g

Ingredients

- 1 lb (450g) fresh mussels, scrubbed and debearded
- 2 tablespoons extra-virgin olive oil
- 3 cloves garlic, minced
- 1 small onion, finely chopped
- 1/2 teaspoon red pepper flakes (optional)
- 1/2 cup dry white wine
- 1 cup canned crushed tomatoes
- 1/2 cup low-sodium vegetable or chicken broth
- Salt and black pepper to taste
- 2 tablespoons chopped fresh parsley
- Lemon wedges, for serving

Directions

- In a large pot, heat the olive oil over medium heat. Add the garlic, onion, and red pepper flakes (if using). Sauté for 3–4 minutes until softened and fragrant.
- Pour in the white wine, scraping the bottom of the pot. Let it simmer for 2 minutes to cook off the alcohol.
- Add the crushed tomatoes and broth. Stir to combine, then bring to a simmer. Season with a pinch of salt and pepper.
- Add the mussels to the pot, cover with a lid, and cook for about 6–8 minutes, or until all the mussels have opened. Discard any that remain closed.
- Stir in fresh parsley and serve immediately with lemon wedges and crusty whole grain bread if desired.

Tips

- Always discard any mussels that do not close when tapped before cooking, and those that do not open after cooking.
- For a heartier meal, serve the mussels over whole wheat pasta or with a side of couscous.

GREEK-STYLE GRILLED OCTOPUS

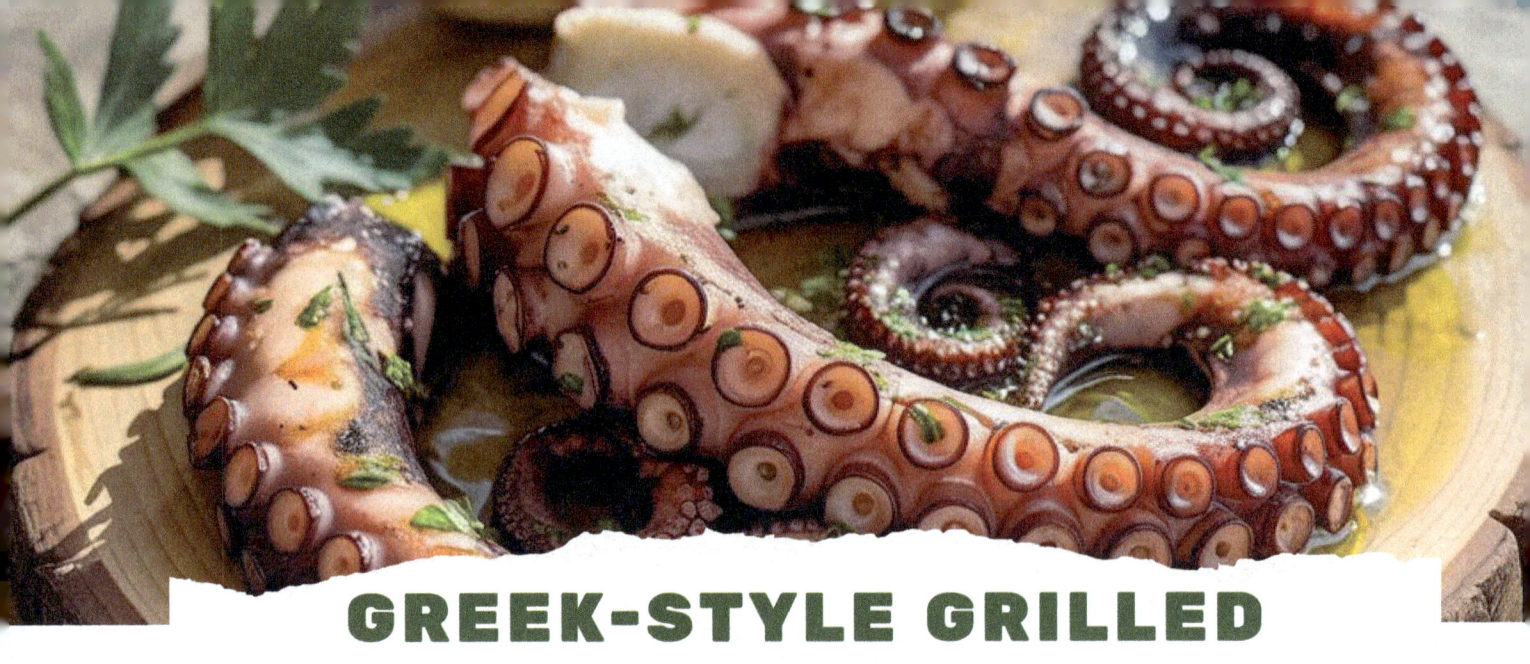

Servings: 4 **Total Time:** 30 Min

Calories: 220 | **Protein:** 25g | **Fat:** 10g | **Carbohydrates:** 4g

Ingredients

- 2 lbs octopus, cleaned
- 1 bay leaf
- 3 garlic cloves, crushed
- 1 lemon, halved
- 1/4 cup extra-virgin olive oil
- 2 tablespoons red wine vinegar
- 1 teaspoon dried oregano
- Salt and black pepper to taste
- Fresh parsley, chopped (for garnish)
- Lemon wedges, for serving

Tips

- Don't skip simmering – it's the key to making the octopus tender before grilling.
- You can prepare the octopus a day ahead and refrigerate it before grilling..
- Serve with a Greek salad or grilled vegetables for a full Mediterranean meal.

Directions

- **Simmer the Octopus:** Place the cleaned octopus in a large pot with enough water to cover. Add bay leaf, garlic, and half a lemon. Bring to a boil, then reduce heat and simmer for about 45–60 minutes, or until the octopus is tender when pierced with a fork.
- **Cool and Prepare:** Remove the octopus from the pot and let it cool slightly. Cut into manageable pieces (tentacles or 2-3 inch segments).
- **Marinate:** In a bowl, whisk together olive oil, red wine vinegar, oregano, salt, and pepper. Toss the octopus in the marinade and let sit for 15–30 minutes.
- **Grill:** Preheat a grill or grill pan over medium-high heat. Grill octopus pieces for 3–4 minutes per side until lightly charred.
- **Serve:** Plate with a drizzle of olive oil, chopped parsley, and lemon wedges on the side.

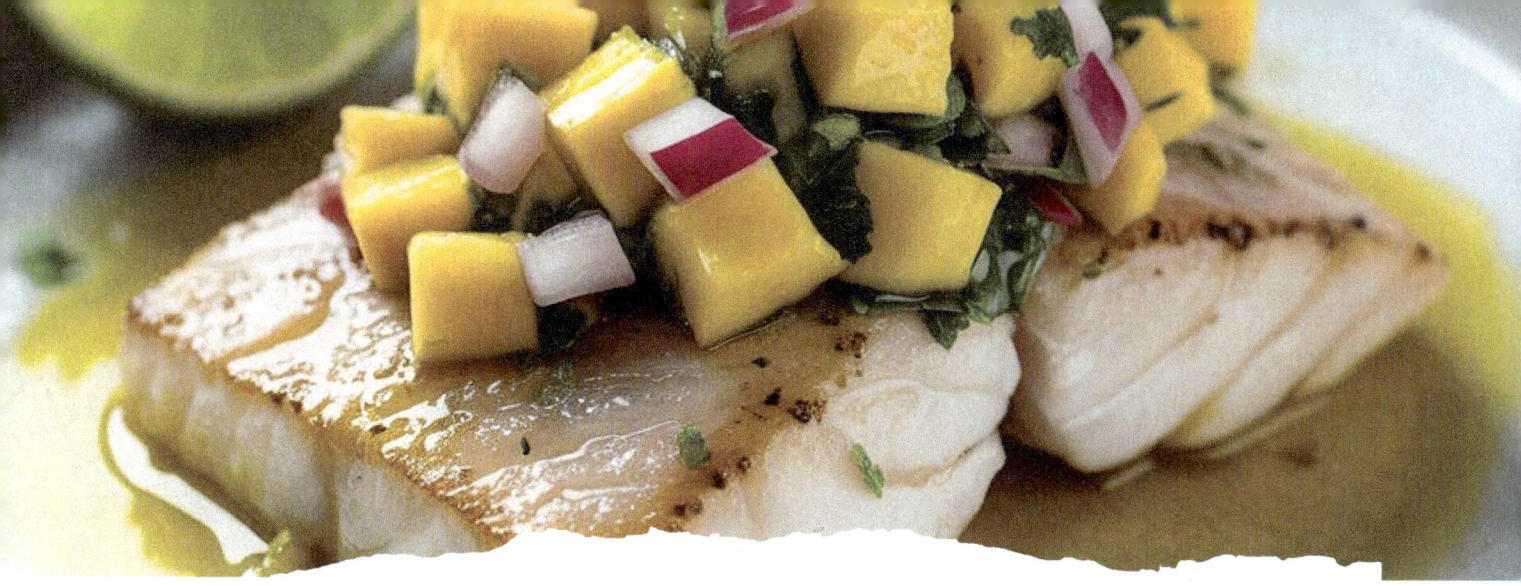

SEARED MAHI MAHI WITH MANGO SALSA

Servings: 2   **Total Time:** 25 Min

Calories: 320 | **Protein:** 32g | **Carbohydrates:** 14g | **Fat:** 16g

Ingredients

For the Mahi Mahi:
- 2 Mahi Mahi fillets (5–6 oz each)
- 1 tablespoon olive oil
- ½ teaspoon sea salt
- ¼ teaspoon black pepper
- ¼ teaspoon paprika
- Juice of ½ lime

For the Mango Salsa:
- 1 ripe mango, peeled and diced
- ¼ red onion, finely chopped
- ½ red bell pepper, diced
- 2 tablespoons fresh cilantro, chopped
- Juice of 1 lime
- Pinch of sea salt
- Optional: ½ jalapeño, finely chopped (for heat)

Directions

- **Prepare the Salsa:** In a bowl, combine the diced mango, red onion, bell pepper, cilantro, lime juice, and salt. Mix well and set aside to allow flavors to blend.
- **Season the Fish:** Pat the Mahi Mahi fillets dry with paper towels. Rub with olive oil, then season with salt, pepper, paprika, and lime juice.
- **Sear the Fish:** Heat a non-stick skillet over medium-high heat. Place the fillets in the pan and cook for 3–4 minutes per side, or until golden and cooked through (fish should flake easily with a fork).
- **Plate and Serve:** Transfer the seared Mahi Mahi to plates and top generously with mango salsa. Serve with a side of greens or brown rice if desired.

Tips

- Use fresh, firm mangoes that aren't overly ripe for the best texture in salsa.
- Can't find Mahi Mahi? Substitute with halibut, cod, or tilapia.
- Add avocado chunks to the salsa for extra creaminess and healthy fats.

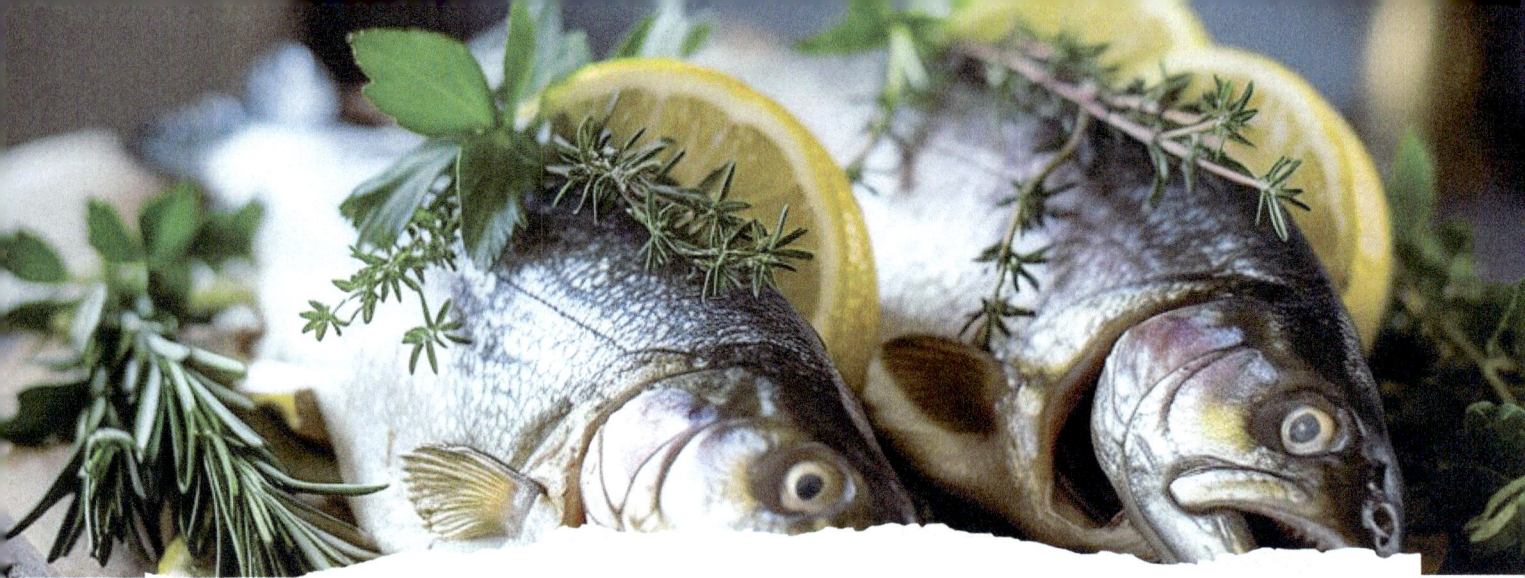

BAKED TROUT WITH HERBS AND LEMON

Servings: 2   **Total Time:** 30 Min

Calories: 320 | **Protein:** 34g | **Fat:** 18g | **Carbohydrates:** 3g

Ingredients

- 2 whole trout, cleaned and gutted
- 2 tablespoons olive oil
- 1 lemon, thinly sliced
- 3 cloves garlic, minced
- 4 sprigs fresh parsley
- 2 sprigs fresh rosemary
- 2 sprigs fresh thyme
- Salt and black pepper to taste

Tips

- For crispier skin, broil the trout for the last 2 minutes of baking.
- Pair with a side of roasted vegetables or a light quinoa salad.
- Don't overcook—trout is delicate and best when just done.
- Fresh herbs work best, but dried herbs can be used in a pinch.

Directions

- Preheat your oven to 375°F (190°C).
- Rinse the trout under cold water and pat dry with paper towels.
- Rub the inside and outside of each fish with olive oil, salt, and pepper.
- Stuff each trout with slices of lemon, garlic, and fresh herbs.
- Place the trout on a baking sheet lined with parchment paper or foil.
- Arrange extra lemon slices on top of the fish for extra flavor and presentation.
- Bake for 20–25 minutes, or until the flesh is opaque and flakes easily with a fork.
- Remove from the oven and serve warm with a drizzle of olive oil or a squeeze of fresh lemon.

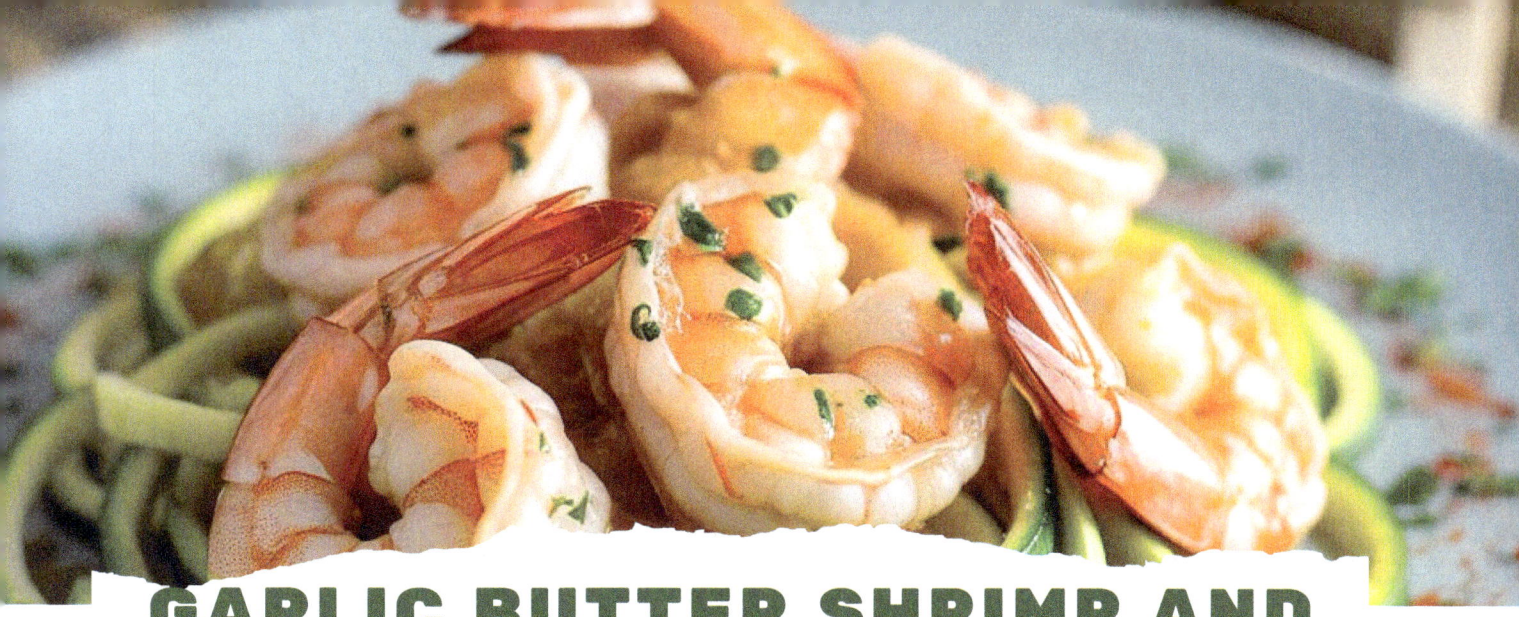

GARLIC BUTTER SHRIMP AND ZOODLES

Servings: 2   **Total Time:** 20 Min

Calories: 260 | **Protein:** 25g | **Carbohydrates:** 7g | **Fat:** 15g

Ingredients

- 1 tablespoon olive oil
- 1 tablespoon unsalted butter
- 2 garlic cloves, minced
- 1/2 teaspoon red pepper flakes (optional)
- 1/2 pound (225g) shrimp, peeled and deveined
- Salt and pepper, to taste
- 2 medium zucchinis, spiralized
- Juice of 1/2 lemon
- 1 tablespoon chopped fresh parsley

Tips

- Use pre-spiralized zucchini to save time.
- Add a sprinkle of Parmesan for extra flavor.
- For more texture, toss in a few cherry tomatoes or baby spinach at the end.
- Make it spicy by adding more red pepper flakes or a dash of hot sauce.

Directions

- Heat olive oil and butter in a large skillet over medium heat.
- Add minced garlic and red pepper flakes (if using), and sauté for 30 seconds until fragrant.
- Add the shrimp, season with salt and pepper, and cook for 2–3 minutes per side until pink and opaque.
- Remove shrimp and set aside.
- In the same skillet, add the zucchini noodles and cook for 2–3 minutes, tossing gently until just tender (do not overcook).
- Return the shrimp to the pan, add lemon juice, and toss everything together for 1 minute.
- Garnish with fresh parsley and serve immediately.

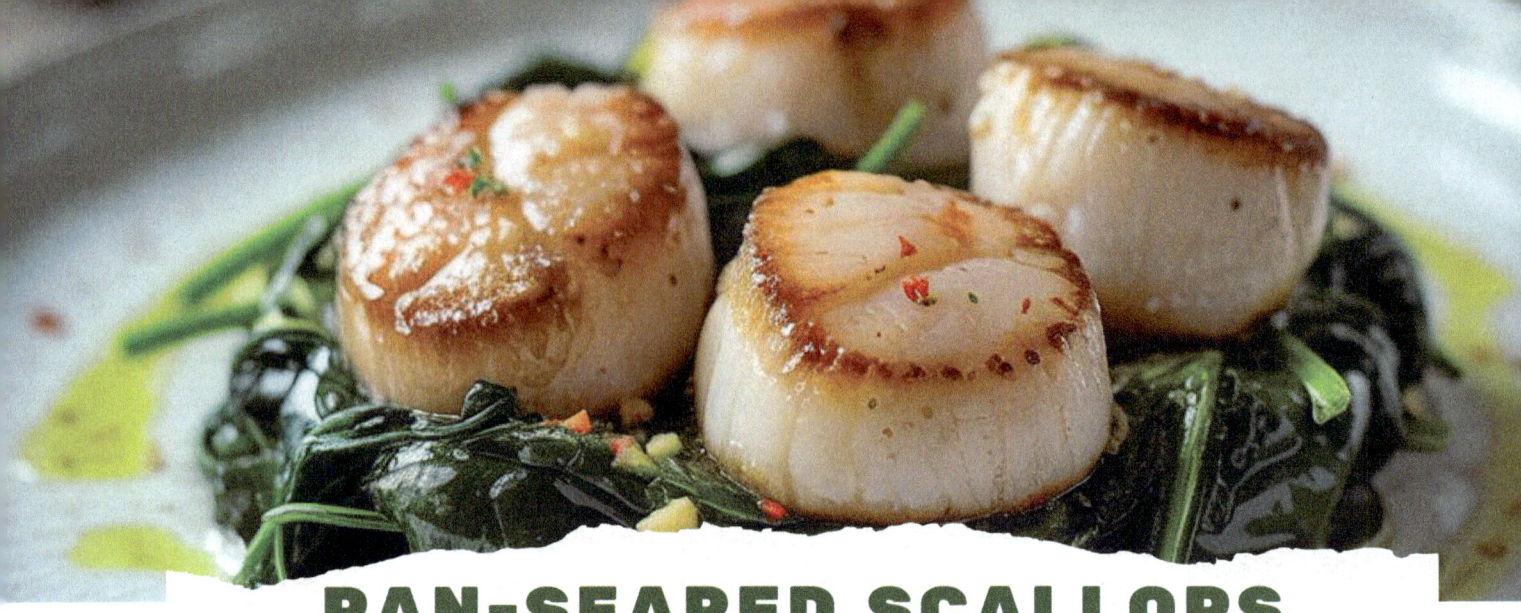

PAN-SEARED SCALLOPS WITH SPINACH

Servings: 2   **Total Time:** 20 Min

Calories: 280 | **Protein:** 24g | **Fat:** 18g | **Carbohydrates:** 5g

Ingredients

- 10–12 large sea scallops, cleaned and patted dry
- 2 tablespoons extra virgin olive oil
- 2 garlic cloves, minced
- 4 cups fresh baby spinach
- 1 tablespoon lemon juice
- Salt and black pepper, to taste
- Optional: pinch of red pepper flakes

Tips

- Make sure the scallops are very dry before searing to get a perfect golden crust.
- Avoid overcooking – scallops cook quickly and turn rubbery if left too long.
- Add a splash of white wine or a dash of butter at the end for extra richness.
- Serve with whole grain couscous or quinoa for a complete Mediterranean meal.

Directions

- **Prep the scallops:** Pat scallops dry with paper towels. Season both sides lightly with salt and pepper.
- **Sear the scallops:** Heat 1 tablespoon olive oil in a non-stick or cast-iron skillet over medium-high heat. When hot, add scallops in a single layer (do not overcrowd). Sear for 2–3 minutes per side until golden brown and slightly opaque in the center. Remove and set aside.
- **Sauté the spinach:** In the same pan, reduce heat to medium. Add the remaining 1 tablespoon of olive oil and minced garlic. Sauté for 30 seconds.
- **Add spinach:** Add spinach and toss gently until just wilted, about 2 minutes. Add lemon juice, red pepper flakes (if using), and a pinch of salt.
- **Serve:** Divide spinach between two plates. Top with seared scallops. Drizzle with any pan juices.

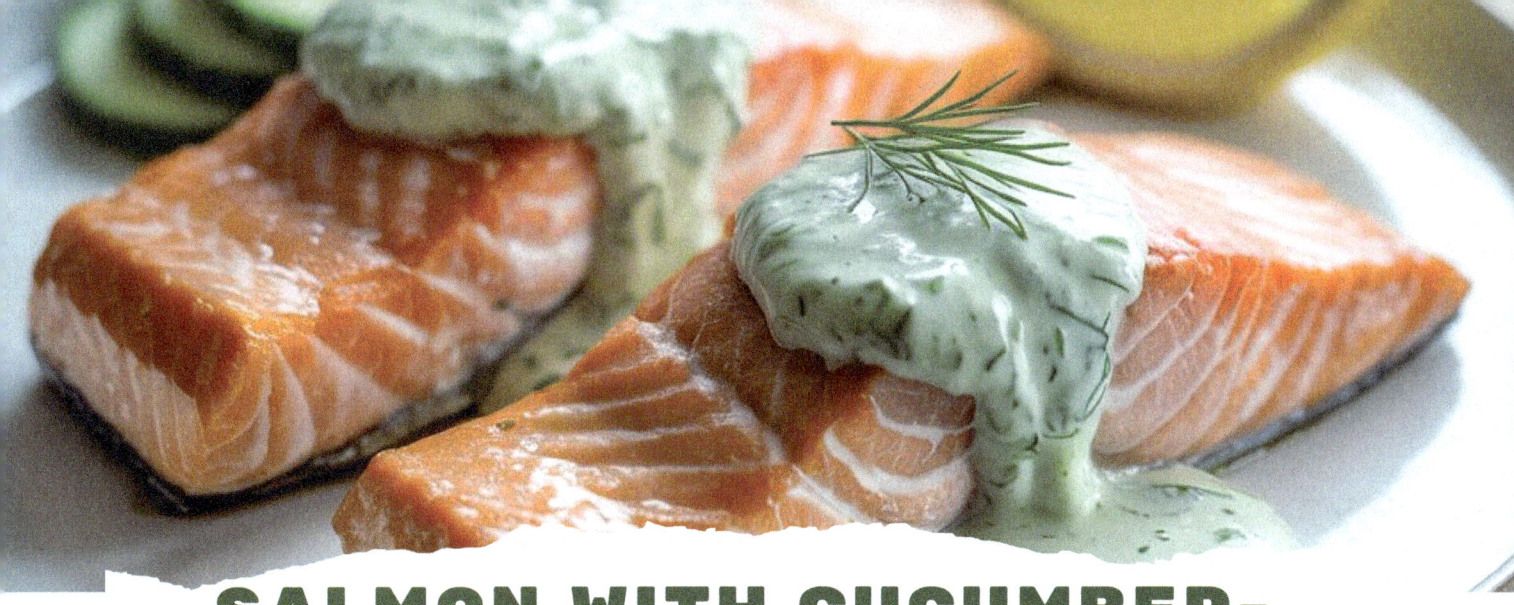

SALMON WITH CUCUMBER-DILL SAUCE

Servings: 2 **Total Time:** 25 Min

Calories: 320 | **Protein:** 30g | **Fat:** 20g | **Carbohydrates:** 4g

Ingredients

- 2 salmon fillets (4–6 oz each)
- 1 tablespoon olive oil
- 1/2 teaspoon sea salt
- 1/4 teaspoon black pepper
- 1/2 teaspoon garlic powder
- 1/2 teaspoon lemon zest

For the Cucumber-Dill Sauce:

- 1/2 cup plain Greek yogurt
- 1/4 cup finely diced cucumber
- 1 tablespoon fresh dill, chopped
- 1 teaspoon lemon juice
- 1 small garlic clove, minced (optional)
- Salt and pepper to taste

Directions

- Preheat your oven to 400°F (200°C). Line a baking sheet with parchment paper.
- Pat the salmon fillets dry and rub with olive oil, salt, pepper, garlic powder, and lemon zest.
- Place the salmon on the baking sheet and bake for 12–15 minutes, or until the salmon flakes easily with a fork.
- While the salmon cooks, make the sauce: in a small bowl, combine Greek yogurt, cucumber, dill, lemon juice, and garlic. Stir well. Season with salt and pepper to taste.
- Serve the salmon warm, topped generously with the cucumber-dill sauce.

Tips

- Use fresh dill for the best flavor, but dried dill can be used in a pinch (use 1 tsp).
- If you don't have an oven, the salmon can be pan-seared for 4–5 minutes per side.
- The cucumber-dill sauce also works well as a dip for veggies or a topping for grilled chicken.

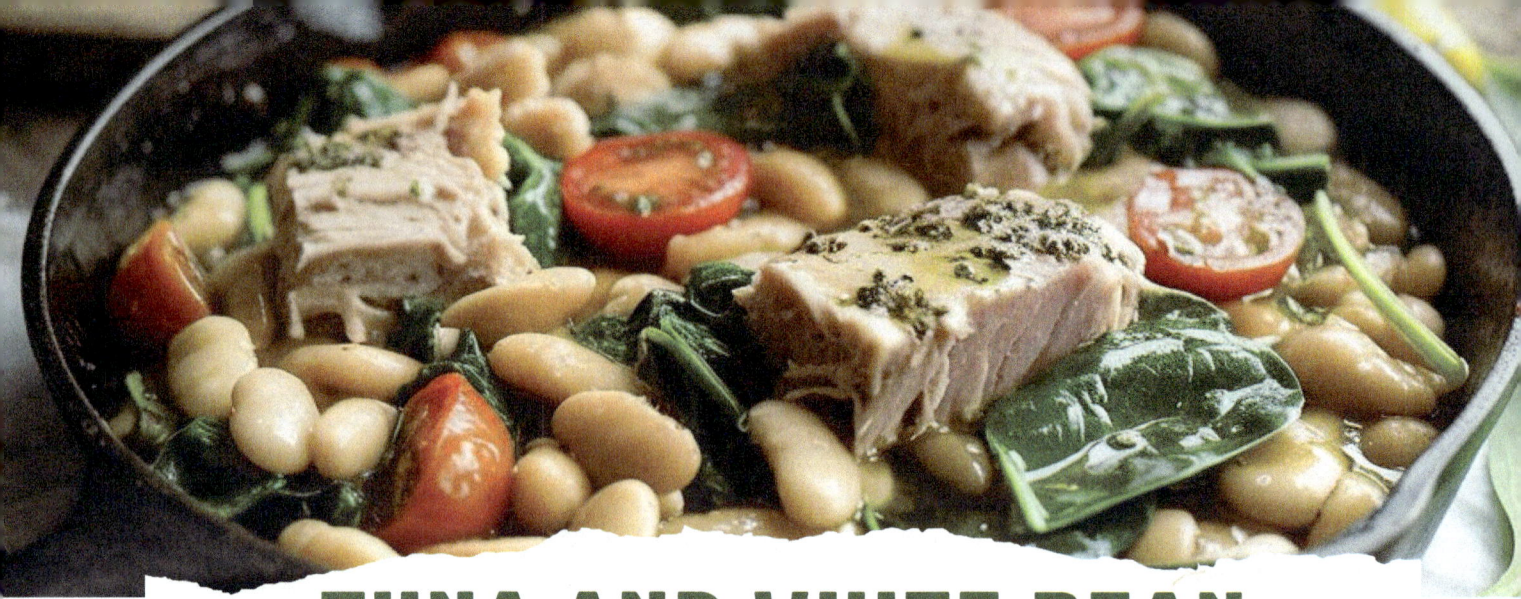

TUNA AND WHITE BEAN SKILLET

Servings: 2 **Total Time:** 20 Min

Calories: 310 | **Protein:** 25g | **Carbohydrates:** 22g | **Fat:** 15g

Ingredients

- 1 tablespoon extra-virgin olive oil
- 1 small red onion, thinly sliced
- 1 garlic clove, minced
- 1 (15 oz) can white beans (cannellini or navy), drained and rinsed
- 1 (5 oz) can tuna in olive oil, drained
- 1 cup cherry tomatoes, halved
- 1 cup baby spinach
- 1 teaspoon dried oregano
- Juice of ½ lemon
- Salt and black pepper, to taste

Directions

- Heat olive oil in a skillet over medium heat.
- Add the red onion and garlic; sauté for 2–3 minutes until fragrant and slightly soft.
- Stir in the cherry tomatoes and cook for another 3–4 minutes until they begin to soften.
- Add the white beans and tuna, gently stirring to combine.
- Toss in the baby spinach and cook until wilted, about 2 minutes.
- Season with oregano, lemon juice, salt, and pepper.
- Serve warm straight from the skillet, with crusty whole grain bread if desired.

Tips

- Use tuna packed in olive oil for a richer flavor, but water-packed works too if you want to cut down fat.
- Add fresh herbs like parsley or basil for extra brightness.
- For a heartier meal, serve with cooked quinoa or farro.

ANCHOVY AND ROASTED PEPPER FLATBREAD

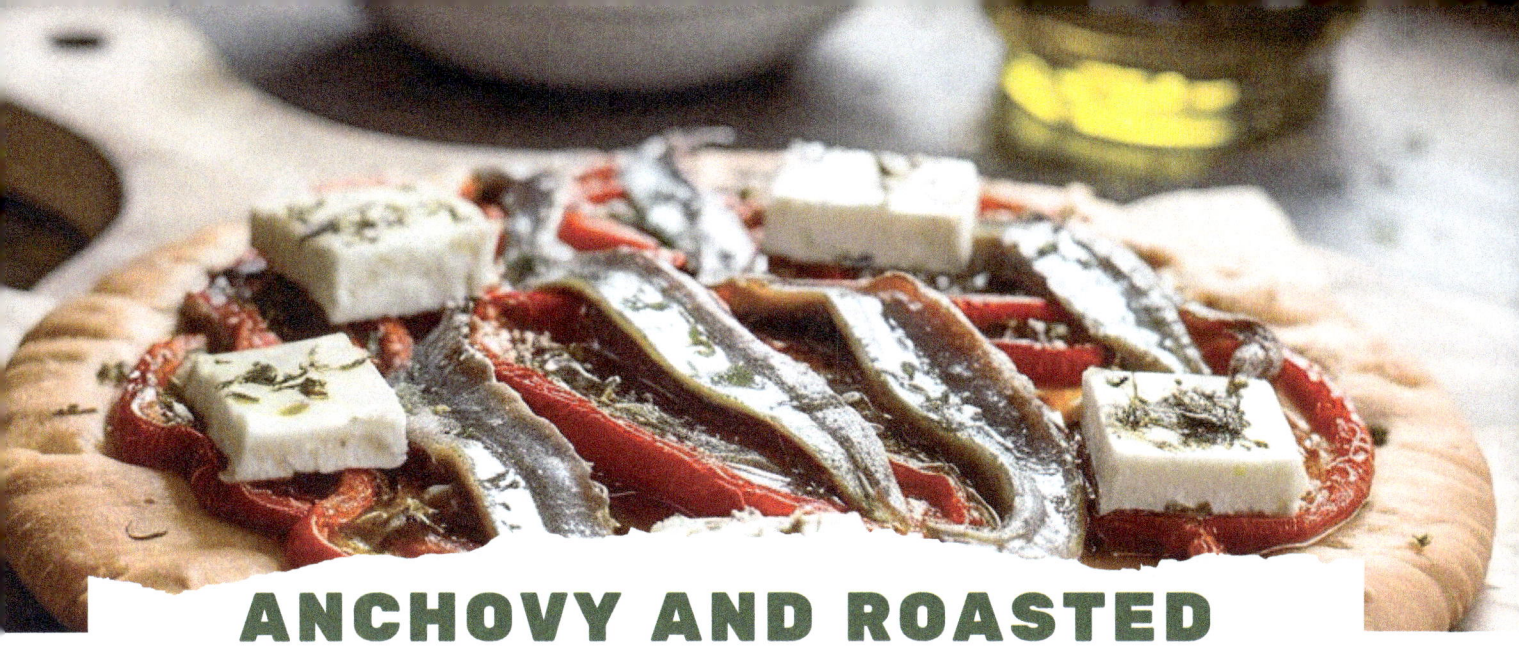

Servings: 2 | **Total Time:** 25 Min

Calories: 280 | **Protein:** 10g | **Carbohydrates:** 22g | **Fat:** 18g

Ingredients

- 1 whole-wheat flatbread or naan
- 1 tablespoon extra-virgin olive oil
- 1 garlic clove, minced
- 1/2 cup roasted red peppers, sliced
- 4–6 anchovy fillets (packed in olive oil), drained
- 1/4 cup crumbled feta cheese
- 1/2 teaspoon dried oregano
- Freshly ground black pepper, to taste
- A handful of arugula or baby spinach (optional, for garnish)

Directions

- Preheat your oven to 400°F (200°C).
- Place the flatbread on a baking sheet. Brush it lightly with olive oil and sprinkle the minced garlic evenly over the top.
- Arrange the roasted red peppers evenly across the flatbread.
- Lay the anchovy fillets on top, spacing them out for even flavor.
- Sprinkle crumbled feta and dried oregano over the flatbread.
- Bake for 10–12 minutes, or until the edges are golden and the cheese is slightly melted.
- Remove from the oven and season with freshly ground black pepper.
- Top with fresh arugula or baby spinach if using. Slice and serve warm.

Tips

- If anchovies are too salty for your taste, soak them in cold water for 5 minutes and pat dry before using.
- You can use store-bought roasted peppers or roast your own at home for extra flavor.
- Swap flatbread with whole wheat pita or cauliflower crust for variation.
- This makes a great appetizer, light lunch, or part of a tapas-style Mediterranean dinner.

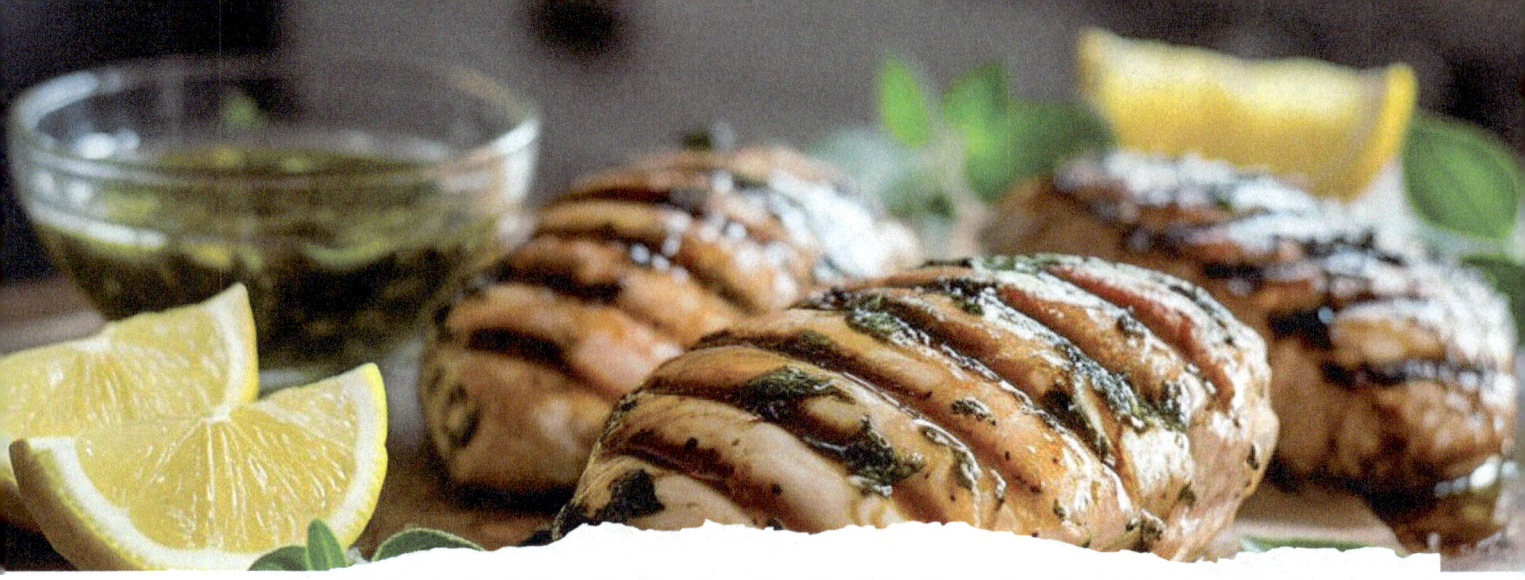

LEMON OREGANO GRILLED CHICKEN

Servings: 2　　**Total Time:** 30 Min

Calories: 280 | **Protein:** 32g | **Carbohydrates:** 2g | **Fat:** 15g

Ingredients

- 2 boneless, skinless chicken breasts
- 2 tablespoons extra-virgin olive oil
- Juice of 1 lemon
- 1 teaspoon lemon zest
- 2 garlic cloves, minced
- 1 tablespoon fresh oregano (or 1 teaspoon dried oregano)
- Salt and black pepper, to taste

Directions

- In a small bowl, whisk together olive oil, lemon juice, lemon zest, garlic, and oregano.
- Season the chicken breasts with salt and pepper on both sides.
- Place the chicken in a resealable bag or shallow dish. Pour the marinade over the chicken, ensuring it's well coated. Let marinate for at least 15 minutes (or up to 4 hours in the fridge for more flavor).
- Preheat your grill or grill pan over medium heat.
- Remove the chicken from the marinade and grill for 6–8 minutes per side, or until fully cooked and golden grill marks appear.
- Let rest for 5 minutes before slicing and serving.

Tips

- For extra juiciness, lightly pound the chicken breasts to even thickness before marinating.
- Serve with a side of Greek salad or roasted vegetables for a complete Mediterranean meal.
- You can cook this on a stovetop grill pan or bake it at 400°F (200°C) for 20–25 minutes if you don't have a grill.

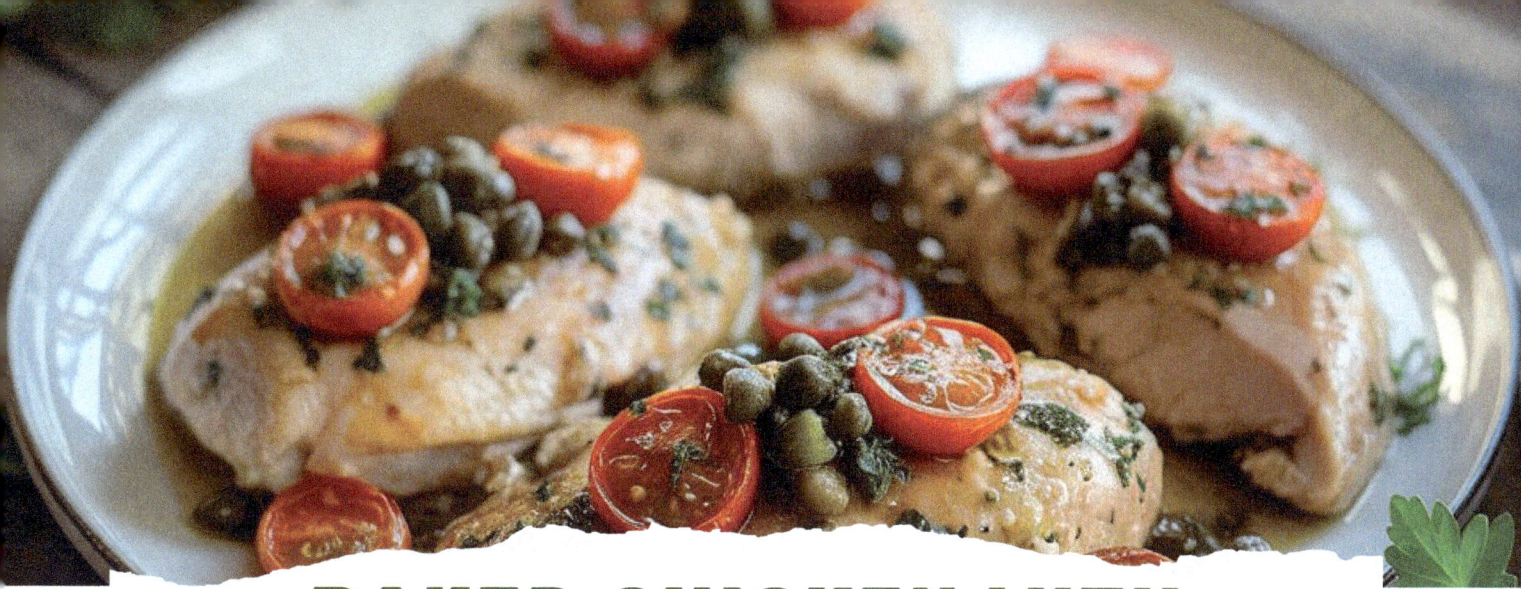

BAKED CHICKEN WITH TOMATOES AND CAPERS

Servings: 4   **Total Time:** 45 Min

Calories: 290 | **Protein:** 30g | **Fat:** 14g | **Carbohydrates:** 8g

Ingredients

- 4 boneless, skinless chicken breasts
- 2 cups cherry tomatoes, halved
- 2 tablespoons capers, drained
- 3 cloves garlic, minced
- 2 tablespoons extra-virgin olive oil
- 1 teaspoon dried oregano
- ½ teaspoon salt
- ¼ teaspoon black pepper
- ¼ cup chopped fresh parsley (optional for garnish)

Directions

- Preheat the oven to 400°F (200°C).
- Place the chicken breasts in a baking dish.
- In a bowl, combine cherry tomatoes, capers, garlic, olive oil, oregano, salt, and pepper. Mix well.
- Pour the tomato mixture over the chicken breasts.
- Bake uncovered for 30–35 minutes, or until the chicken is cooked through and the tomatoes are soft and juicy.
- Garnish with chopped fresh parsley before serving (optional).

Tips

- Use skin-on, bone-in chicken thighs for richer flavor, but adjust the cooking time as needed.
- Serve over brown rice, couscous, or alongside a green salad for a complete meal.
- Add olives or artichoke hearts for extra Mediterranean flair.

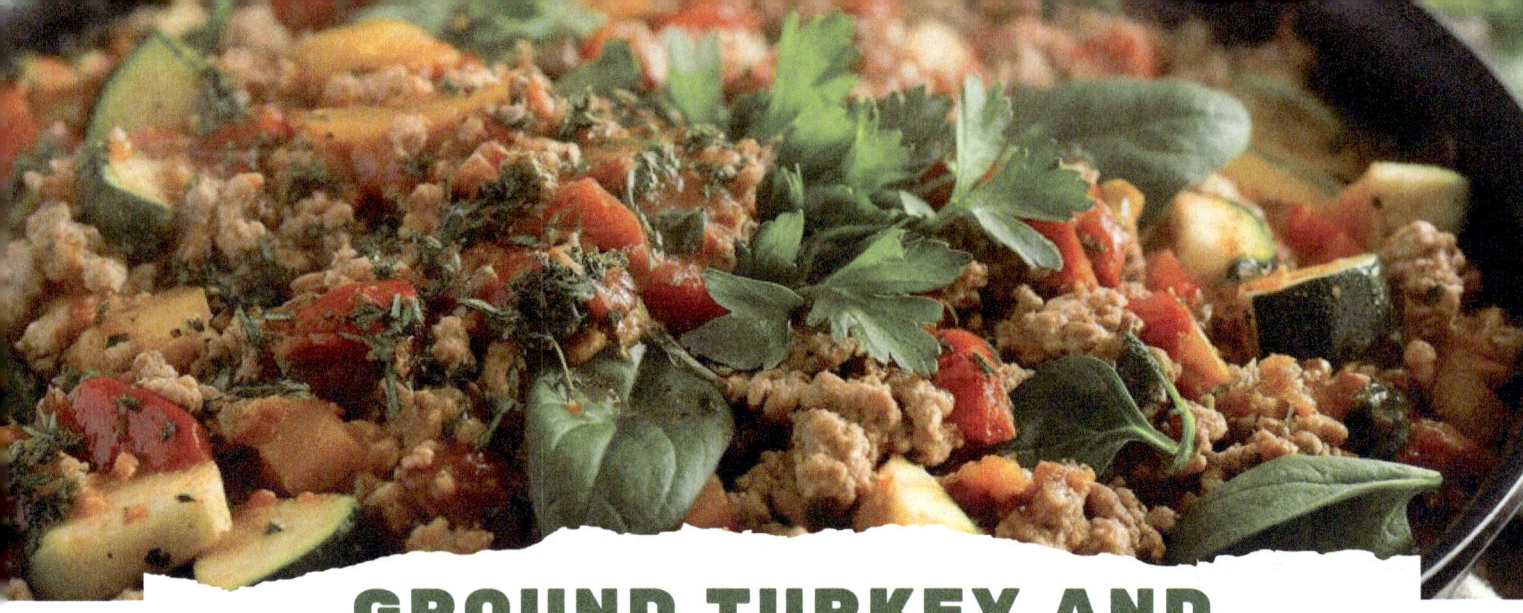

GROUND TURKEY AND VEGGIE SKILLET

Servings: 4 | **Total Time:** 30 Min

Calories: 290 | **Protein:** 28g | **Carbohydrates:** 10g | **Fat:** 16g

Ingredients

- 1 lb (450g) ground turkey
- 2 tablespoons olive oil
- 1 small onion, diced
- 2 garlic cloves, minced
- 1 zucchini, chopped
- 1 red bell pepper, chopped
- 1 cup cherry tomatoes, halved
- 1 cup baby spinach
- 1 teaspoon dried oregano
- 1/2 teaspoon paprika
- Salt and pepper to taste
- Fresh parsley for garnish

Directions

- Heat olive oil in a large skillet over medium heat.
- Add diced onion and cook for 2–3 minutes until softened.
- Stir in garlic and cook for 30 seconds until fragrant.
- Add ground turkey, breaking it up with a spoon. Cook until browned and no longer pink, about 6–8 minutes.
- Add zucchini, bell pepper, and cherry tomatoes. Cook for another 5–7 minutes, stirring occasionally.
- Stir in spinach, oregano, paprika, salt, and pepper. Cook for 2–3 more minutes until the spinach wilts and veggies are tender.
- Garnish with fresh parsley and serve warm.

Tips

- Use pre-chopped vegetables to save time.
- Add a sprinkle of feta cheese for extra flavor.
- Pairs well with brown rice or quinoa for a heartier meal.

CHICKEN WITH ARTICHOKES AND OLIVES

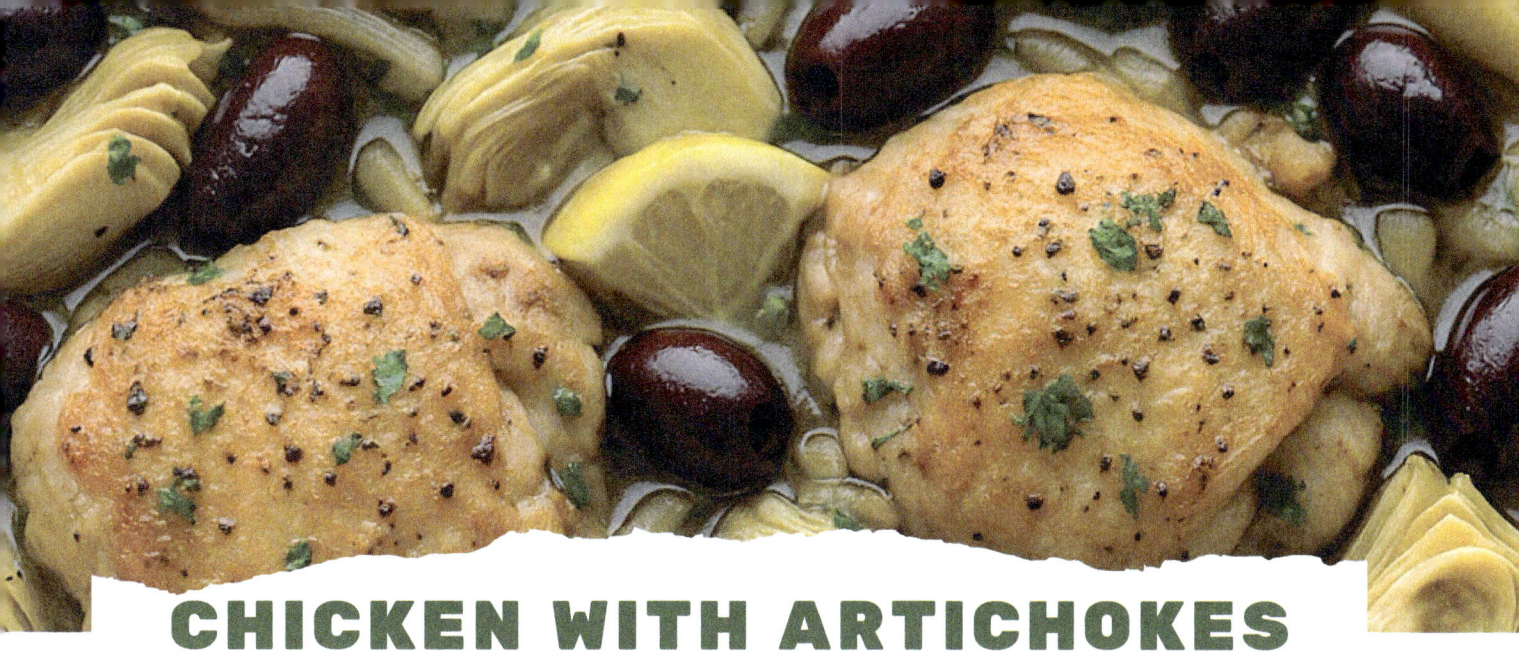

Servings: 4   **Total Time:** 35 Min

Calories: 290 | **Protein:** 27g | **Fat:** 16g | **Carbohydrates:** 7g

Ingredients

- 4 boneless, skinless chicken thighs (or breasts)
- 1 tablespoon extra-virgin olive oil
- 1 small onion, thinly sliced
- 2 garlic cloves, minced
- 1 teaspoon dried oregano
- 1/2 cup low-sodium chicken broth
- 1 can (14 oz) artichoke hearts, drained and halved
- 1/3 cup Kalamata olives, pitted and halved
- Juice of 1/2 lemon
- Salt and pepper to taste
- Fresh parsley (optional, for garnish)

Directions

- Heat the olive oil in a large skillet over medium heat. Add the chicken and season with salt, pepper, and oregano. Cook for 5–6 minutes on each side until golden and cooked through. Remove and set aside.
- In the same pan, sauté the onion for 2–3 minutes until soft. Add garlic and cook for another 30 seconds.
- Pour in the chicken broth, scraping the bottom of the pan to release any browned bits.
- Add the artichoke hearts and olives, then return the chicken to the skillet. Cover and simmer on low for 10 minutes.
- Squeeze in the lemon juice and stir gently.
- Garnish with fresh parsley and serve warm.

Tips

- For extra flavor, marinate the chicken in olive oil, lemon, and garlic 30 minutes before cooking.
- You can substitute green olives if you prefer a milder taste.
- Serve with whole grains like quinoa, couscous, or brown rice for a complete Mediterranean meal.

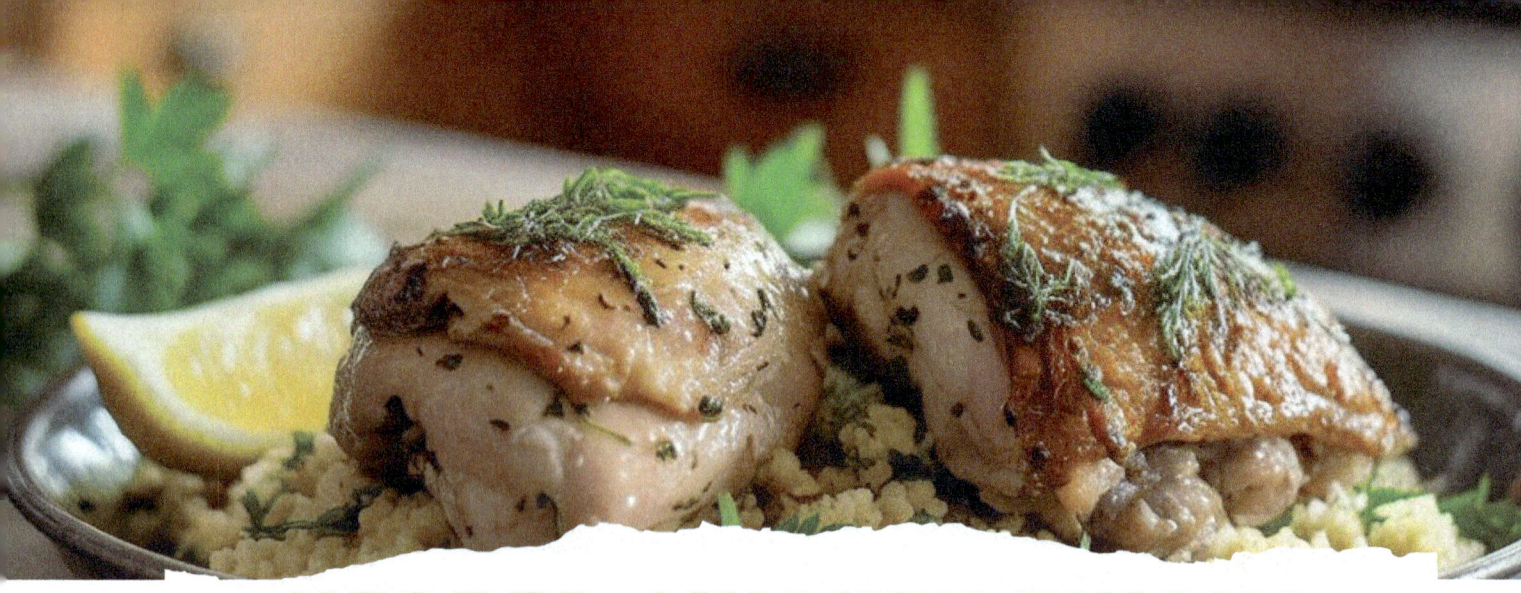

HERBED CHICKEN THIGHS WITH COUSCOUS

Servings: 4 **Total Time:** 35 Min

Calories: 420 | **Protein:** 30g | **Carbohydrates:** 28g | **Fat:** 21g

Ingredients

For the Chicken:
- 4 bone-in, skin-on chicken thighs
- 2 tablespoons olive oil
- 1 teaspoon dried oregano
- 1 teaspoon dried thyme
- 1 teaspoon garlic powder
- ½ teaspoon paprika
- Salt and pepper to taste

For the Couscous:
- 1 cup whole wheat couscous
- 1¼ cups low-sodium chicken broth or water
- 1 tablespoon olive oil
- ½ teaspoon salt
- ¼ cup chopped fresh parsley
- Juice of ½ lemon

Directions

- Preheat the oven to 400°F (200°C).
- Season the chicken thighs with oregano, thyme, garlic powder, paprika, salt, and pepper.
- Heat 2 tablespoons olive oil in a large oven-safe skillet over medium heat.
- Sear the chicken thighs skin-side down for 4–5 minutes until golden. Flip and cook another 3 minutes.
- Transfer skillet to the oven and bake for 20–25 minutes, until internal temperature reaches 165°F (74°C).
- While the chicken bakes, prepare the couscous: bring broth (or water), olive oil, and salt to a boil in a pot.
- Stir in couscous, remove from heat, cover, and let sit for 5 minutes. Fluff with a fork.
- Stir in parsley and lemon juice.
- Serve chicken over couscous and drizzle with pan juices.

Tips

- Substitute boneless thighs if preferred, but reduce oven time by 5–7 minutes.
- Add chopped cherry tomatoes or steamed veggies to couscous for more color and nutrition.
- For crispier chicken skin, broil for 1–2 minutes after baking.

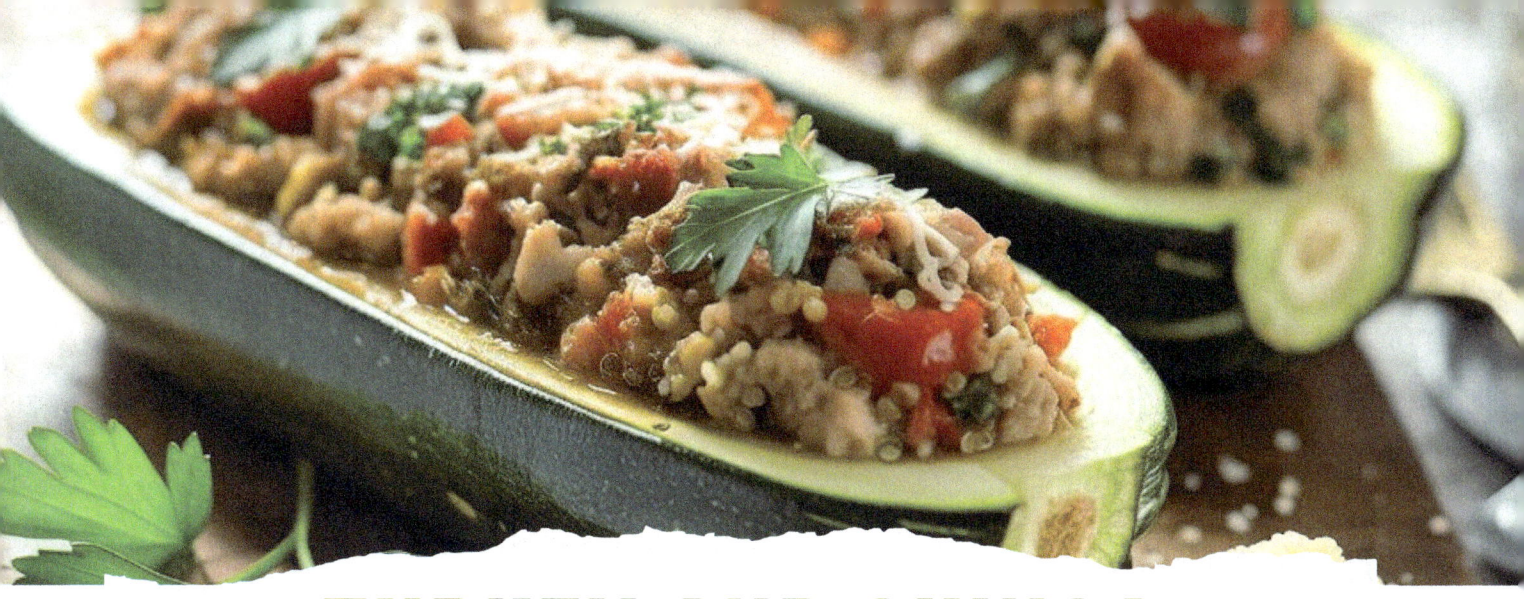

TURKEY AND QUINOA STUFFED ZUCCHINI

Servings: 4 **Total Time:** 45 Min

Calories: 220 | **Protein:** 20g | **Carbohydrates:** 12g | **Fat:** 10g

Ingredients

- 4 medium zucchini
- 1 tablespoon olive oil
- 1 small onion, finely chopped
- 2 cloves garlic, minced
- 1/2 pound ground turkey
- 1/2 cup cooked quinoa
- 1/2 cup diced tomatoes (canned or fresh)
- 1/4 cup chopped fresh parsley
- 1/4 teaspoon dried oregano
- Salt and pepper to taste
- 1/4 cup grated Parmesan cheese

Directions

- Preheat your oven to 375°F (190°C).
- Cut each zucchini in half lengthwise and scoop out the center using a spoon, leaving a 1/4-inch shell. Set aside the scooped flesh.
- In a skillet, heat olive oil over medium heat. Sauté onion and garlic until fragrant and soft, about 3–4 minutes.
- Add ground turkey and cook until browned, breaking it apart as it cooks.
- Stir in the chopped zucchini flesh, cooked quinoa, diced tomatoes, oregano, salt, and pepper. Cook for another 5–7 minutes.
- Remove from heat and stir in chopped parsley.
- Spoon the turkey-quinoa mixture into the hollowed zucchini halves. Place them in a baking dish.
- Sprinkle with Parmesan cheese if desired.
- Cover with foil and bake for 25–30 minutes, until the zucchini is tender. Remove foil for the last 5 minutes if you want a lightly browned top.

Tips

- For added flavor, try mixing in chopped sun-dried tomatoes or olives.
- You can use ground chicken instead of turkey.
- Make it vegetarian by swapping turkey with lentils or more quinoa.
- These stuffed zucchinis freeze well—just wrap and reheat in the oven or microwave.

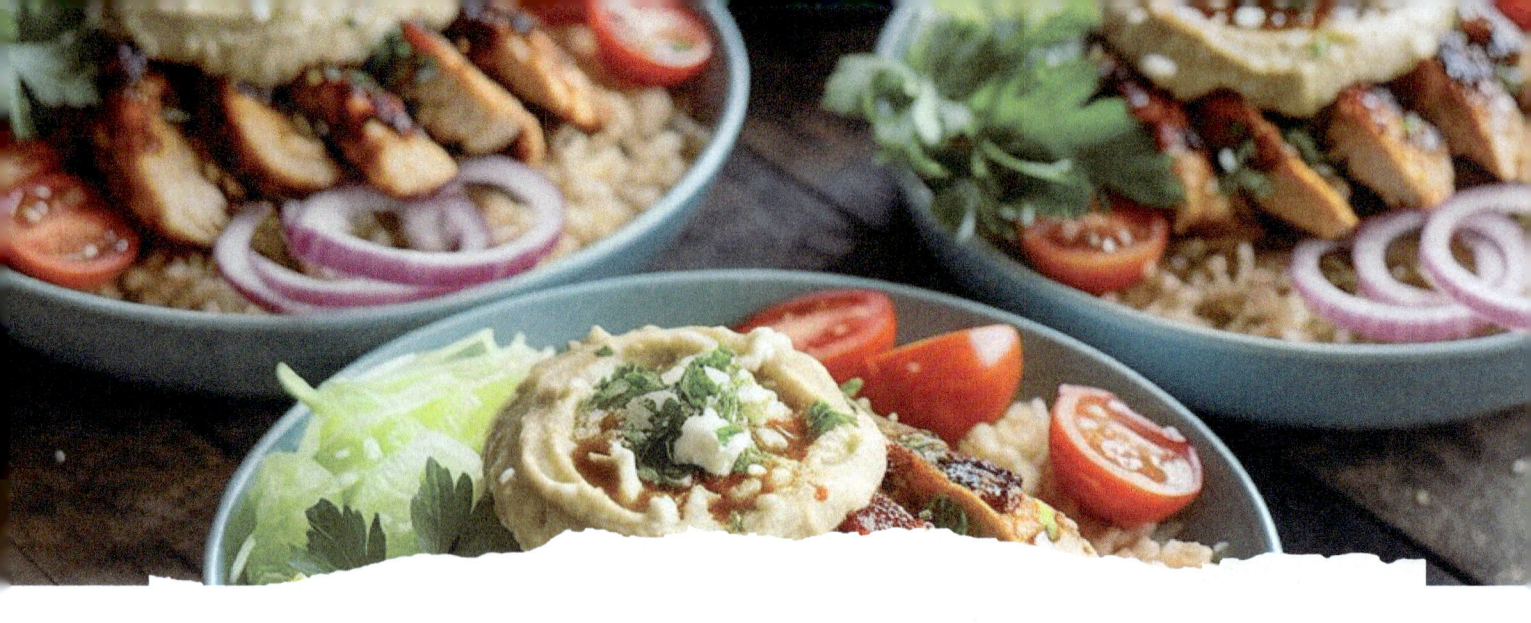

CHICKEN SHAWARMA BOWLS

Servings: 4　　**Total Time:** 35 Min

Calories: 470 | **Protein:** 38g | **Carbohydrates:** 30g | **Fat:** 22g

Ingredients

For the Chicken Marinade:
- 1 ½ lbs boneless, skinless chicken thighs
- 3 tablespoons plain Greek yogurt
- 2 tablespoons olive oil
- 1 tablespoon lemon juice
- 3 garlic cloves, minced
- 1 teaspoon ground cumin
- 1 teaspoon smoked paprika
- ½ teaspoon turmeric
- ½ teaspoon ground cinnamon
- ½ teaspoon ground coriander
- ½ teaspoon salt
- ¼ teaspoon black pepper

For the Bowls:
- 2 cups cooked brown rice or couscous
- 1 cup chopped cucumber
- 1 cup cherry tomatoes, halved
- ½ red onion, thinly sliced
- 1 cup shredded lettuce or mixed greens
- ½ cup hummus
- ¼ cup crumbled feta cheese (optional)
- Fresh parsley, chopped (for garnish)
- Lemon wedges (for serving)

Directions

- Marinate the chicken: In a large bowl, mix Greek yogurt, olive oil, lemon juice, garlic, and all spices. Add chicken thighs and coat well. Cover and refrigerate for at least 20 minutes (or up to overnight for deeper flavor).
- Cook the chicken: Heat a skillet or grill pan over medium-high heat. Cook the marinated chicken for 5–6 minutes per side, or until fully cooked and slightly charred. Let rest for 5 minutes, then slice.
- Assemble the bowls: Divide the cooked rice or couscous into 4 bowls. Top each with chicken, cucumber, cherry tomatoes, red onion, and greens. Add a dollop of hummus and sprinkle with feta, if using.
- Garnish and serve: Sprinkle chopped parsley on top and serve with a wedge of lemon. Enjoy warm or at room temperature.

Tips

- Swap chicken thighs for breasts if you prefer leaner meat.
- Use pre-cooked brown rice or frozen quinoa to save time.
- Add pickled onions or olives for extra tang.
- Make it vegetarian by replacing the chicken with roasted chickpeas or grilled halloumi.
- These bowls keep well in the fridge – great for meal prep!

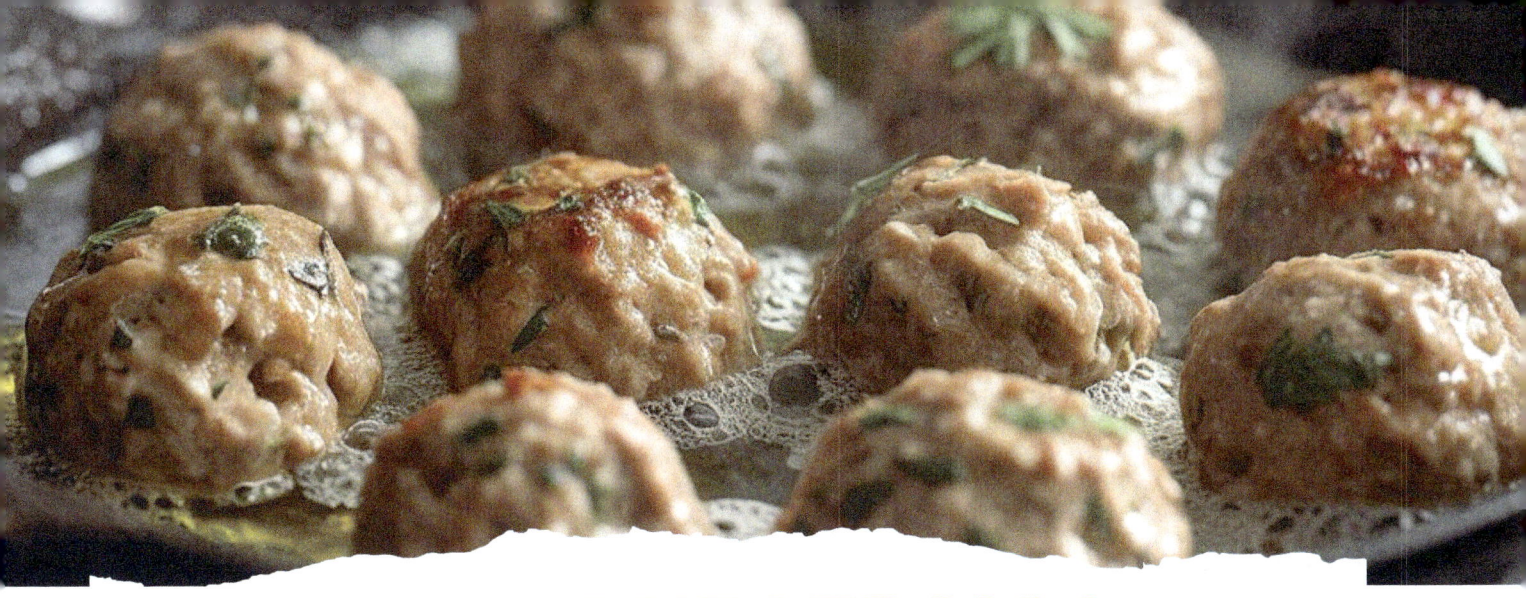

GREEK MEATBALLS (KEFTEDES)

Servings: 4 **Total Time:** 35 Min

Calories: 320 | **Protein:** 22g | **Carbohydrates:** 10g | **Fat:** 22g

Ingredients

- 1 lb (450g) ground beef or lamb
- 1 small onion, finely grated
- 2 cloves garlic, minced
- ¼ cup fresh parsley, chopped
- 1 tbsp fresh mint or 1 tsp dried mint
- 1 tsp dried oregano
- ½ cup breadcrumbs
- 1 egg
- Salt and pepper to taste
- Olive oil, for frying

Directions

- In a large bowl, combine ground meat, grated onion, garlic, parsley, mint, oregano, breadcrumbs, egg, salt, and pepper. Mix until well combined.
- Roll the mixture into small meatballs (about 1½ inches in diameter).
- Heat olive oil in a skillet over medium heat.
- Cook the meatballs in batches, turning occasionally, until browned and cooked through (about 10–12 minutes total).
- Remove and drain on paper towels. Serve warm with a side of tzatziki or a fresh salad.

Tips

- For a lighter version, you can bake the meatballs at 400°F (200°C) for 18–20 minutes instead of frying.
- These pair wonderfully with whole-grain pita, roasted vegetables, or couscous.
- You can freeze uncooked meatballs for up to 2 months. Thaw before cooking.

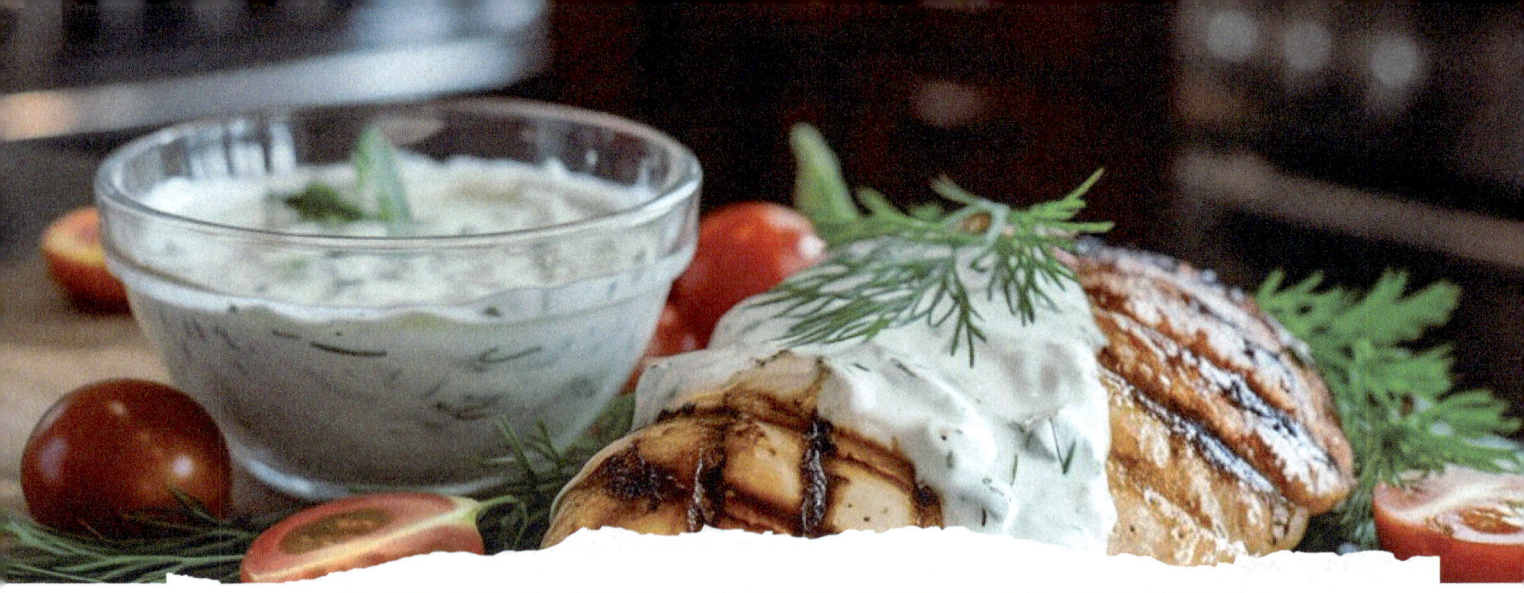

GRILLED CHICKEN WITH TZATZIKI

Servings: 2　　**Total Time:** 30 Min

Calories: 320 | **Protein:** 35g | **Fat:** 18g | **Carbohydrates:** 4g

Ingredients

For the Chicken:
- 2 boneless, skinless chicken breasts
- 2 tablespoons olive oil
- Juice of 1 lemon
- 2 garlic cloves, minced
- 1 teaspoon dried oregano
- Salt and black pepper to taste

For the Tzatziki Sauce:
- ½ cup plain Greek yogurt
- ¼ cucumber, grated and squeezed dry
- 1 garlic clove, minced
- 1 tablespoon fresh dill or mint, chopped
- 1 tablespoon olive oil
- 1 teaspoon lemon juice
- Salt to taste

Directions

- Marinate the Chicken: In a bowl, mix olive oil, lemon juice, garlic, oregano, salt, and pepper. Add chicken breasts and coat well. Let marinate for 15–20 minutes (or longer if you have time).
- Make the Tzatziki: In another bowl, combine yogurt, grated cucumber, garlic, dill or mint, olive oil, and lemon juice. Stir well and season with salt. Chill in the fridge while the chicken cooks.
- Grill the Chicken: Heat a grill pan or outdoor grill over medium heat. Grill chicken for 5–7 minutes per side, or until fully cooked and juices run clear.
- Serve: Let the chicken rest for 2 minutes, then slice and serve with a generous spoonful of tzatziki on top or on the side.

Tips

- Serve the sliced chicken and tzatziki over rice, couscous, or a bed of greens for a quick Mediterranean bowl.
- Pair with pita, grilled veggies, or a Greek salad for a more complete meal.
- Let the sauce sit in the fridge for at least 15 minutes to let the flavors meld together.

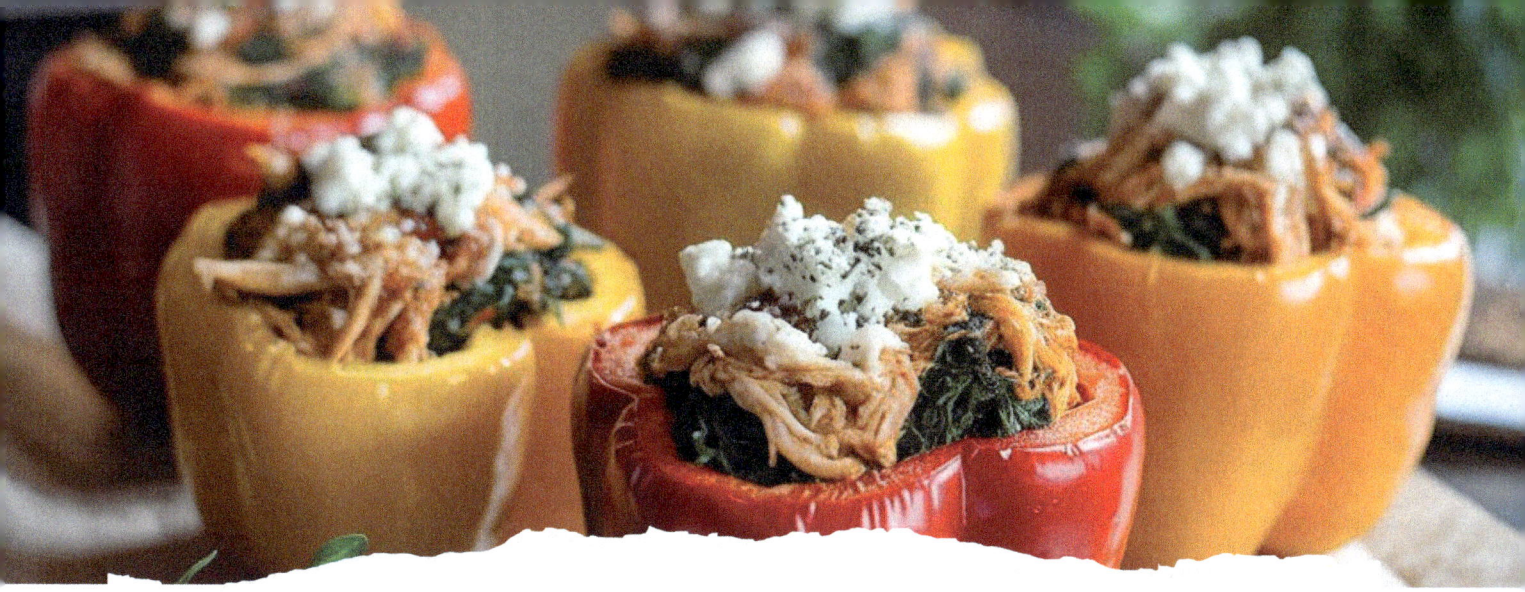

CHICKEN AND SPINACH STUFFED PEPPERS

Servings: 4 **Total Time:** 45 Min

Calories: 320 | **Protein:** 28g | **Carbohydrates:** 22g | **Fat:** 14g

Ingredients

- 4 large bell peppers (red or yellow), tops cut off and seeds removed
- 1 tablespoon olive oil
- 1 small onion, diced
- 2 garlic cloves, minced
- 2 cups cooked chicken breast, shredded
- 2 cups fresh spinach, chopped
- 1 cup cooked brown rice or quinoa
- 1 teaspoon dried oregano
- ½ teaspoon black pepper
- Salt to taste
- ½ cup crumbled feta cheese
- ½ cup shredded mozzarella or part-skim cheese (optional for topping)

Directions

- Preheat oven to 375°F (190°C).
- In a large skillet, heat olive oil over medium heat. Sauté onions for 2–3 minutes until soft, then add garlic and cook for another 30 seconds.
- Add spinach and cook until wilted. Stir in the shredded chicken, cooked rice (or quinoa), oregano, salt, and pepper. Remove from heat and mix in feta cheese if using.
- Spoon the mixture evenly into the hollowed-out bell peppers.
- Place stuffed peppers in a baking dish. If desired, sprinkle mozzarella on top of each.
- Cover with foil and bake for 30 minutes. Remove foil and bake an additional 5–10 minutes to brown the tops.
- Let cool for a few minutes before serving.

Tips

- Swap chicken with canned tuna, cooked lentils, or chickpeas for variety.
- Use pre-cooked rotisserie chicken for faster prep.
- Make ahead and store in the fridge for up to 3 days – just reheat and enjoy.
- Add fresh herbs like parsley or basil for extra flavor.

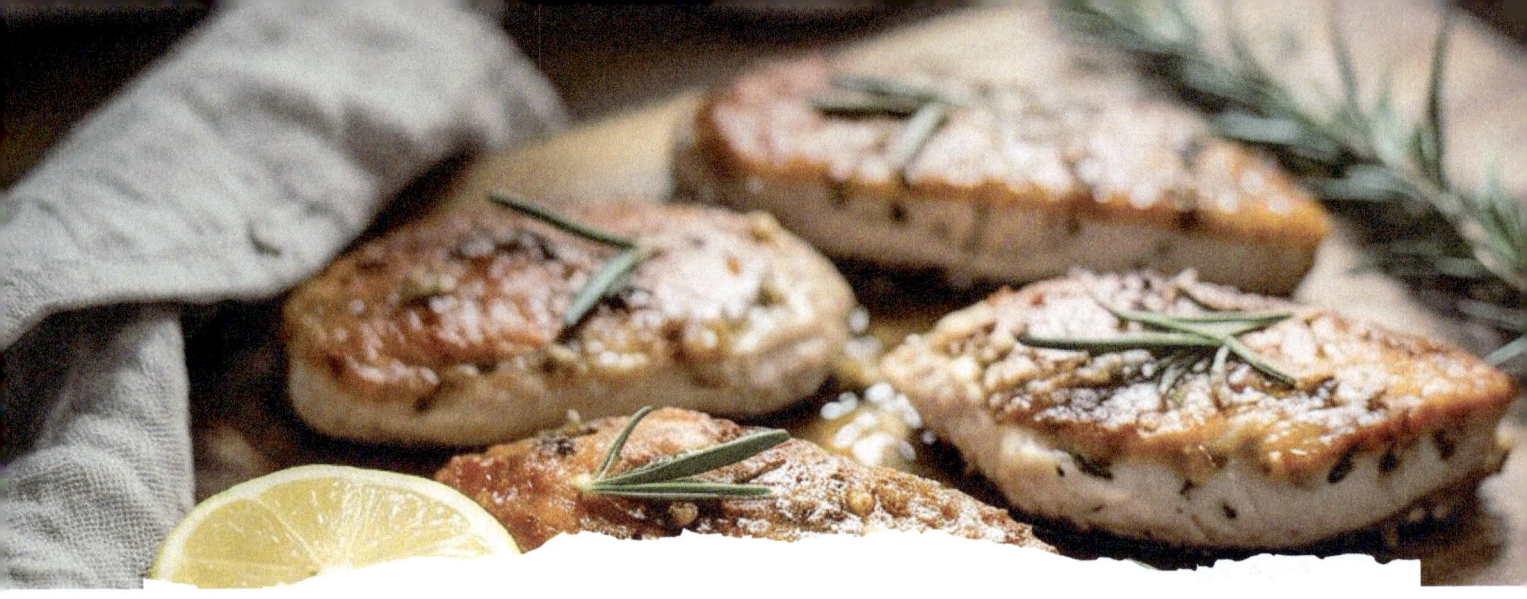

ROSEMARY GARLIC TURKEY CUTLETS

Servings: 2   **Total Time:** 25 Min

Calories: 240 | **Protein:** 32g | **Fat:** 10g | **Carbohydrates:** 1g

Ingredients

- 2 turkey breast cutlets (about 4–5 oz each)
- 1 tablespoon olive oil
- 2 garlic cloves, minced
- 1 teaspoon fresh rosemary, finely chopped (or ½ tsp dried)
- ½ teaspoon salt
- ¼ teaspoon black pepper
- Juice of ½ lemon

Directions

- Pat the turkey cutlets dry with a paper towel.
- In a small bowl, mix the olive oil, minced garlic, rosemary, salt, and pepper.
- Rub the mixture evenly over both sides of the turkey cutlets.
- Heat a nonstick or cast-iron skillet over medium heat.
- Cook the cutlets for 3–4 minutes on each side, or until golden brown and fully cooked (internal temp should reach 165°F).
- Squeeze lemon juice over the cutlets before serving for added brightness.

Tips

- Fresh rosemary gives the best flavor, but dried will work in a pinch.
- Pair with a simple Mediterranean side like roasted vegetables, quinoa, or a tomato-cucumber salad.
- Marinate the cutlets ahead of time (up to 12 hours) for extra flavor and tenderness.

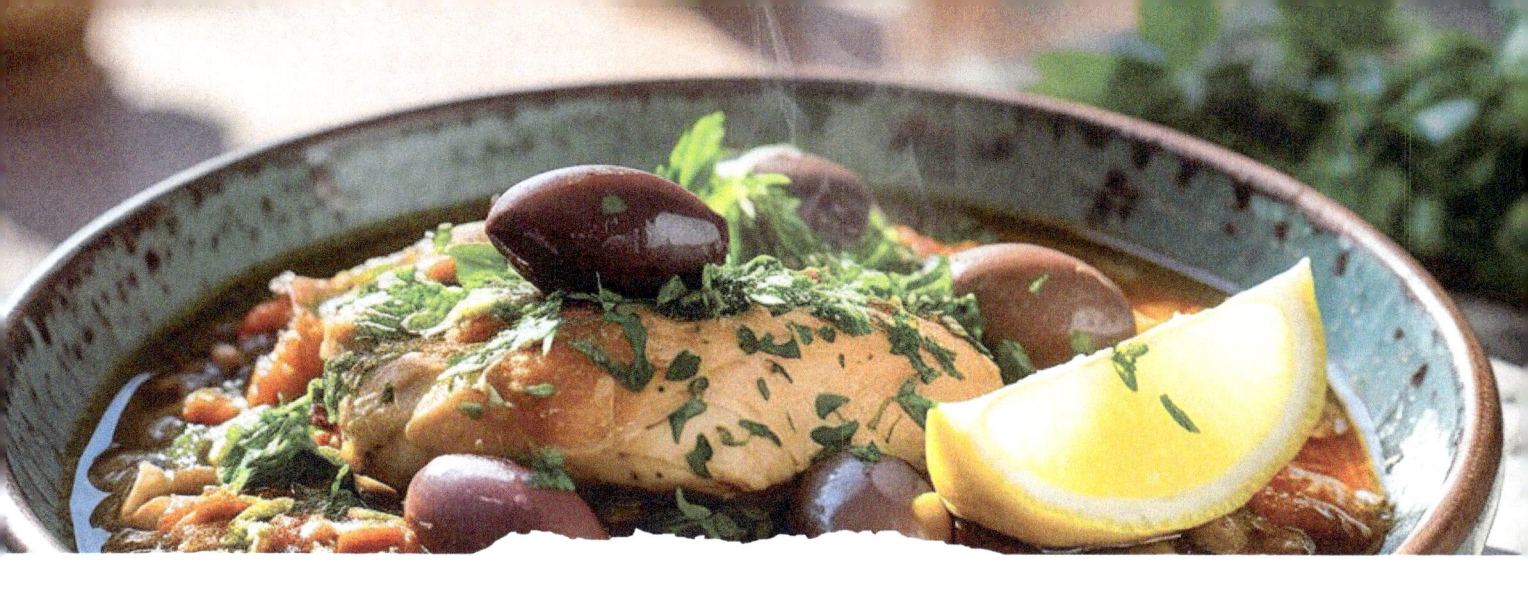

MEDITERRANEAN CHICKEN AND LENTILS

Servings: 4 **Total Time:** 40 Min

Calories: 380 | **Protein:** 40g | **Carbs:** 30g | **Fat:** 10g

Ingredients

- 4 boneless, skinless chicken breasts
- 1 cup dried lentils, rinsed
- 1 medium onion, chopped
- 2 cloves garlic, minced
- 1 can (14.5 oz) diced tomatoes, drained
- 1/2 cup low-sodium chicken broth
- 1 tablespoon olive oil
- 1 teaspoon ground cumin
- 1 teaspoon ground coriander
- 1 teaspoon dried oregano
- 1/2 teaspoon ground cinnamon
- Salt and pepper to taste
- 1/2 cup Kalamata olives, pitted and sliced
- 1/4 cup fresh parsley, chopped
- 1 tablespoon lemon juice
- Zest of 1 lemon

Tips

- You can use any lentils you prefer, but green or brown lentils hold their shape best in this dish.
- If you prefer, you can swap out the chicken breasts for thighs or even use grilled chicken for a different flavor.
- For a vegetarian version, replace the chicken with extra vegetables like zucchini or eggplant and add more olives for a savory flavor.
- This dish can be made ahead and stored in the fridge for up to 3 days. Reheat it gently before serving.

Directions

- Cook the Lentils: In a medium pot, add lentils and cover with water. Bring to a boil, reduce the heat, and simmer for about 20-25 minutes, or until tender but still firm. Drain and set aside.
- Cook the Chicken: Heat olive oil in a large skillet over medium heat. Season the chicken breasts with salt, pepper, cumin, coriander, and oregano. Add the chicken to the skillet and cook for 6-7 minutes per side, or until browned and fully cooked through. Remove the chicken from the skillet and set aside.
- Prepare the Base: In the same skillet, add the onion and garlic. Cook for 3-4 minutes, until softened. Add the cinnamon and cook for another 30 seconds, until fragrant.
- Combine the Ingredients: Add the diced tomatoes and chicken broth to the skillet, stirring to combine. Bring to a simmer and let cook for 5 minutes.
- Add the Lentils: Add the cooked lentils to the skillet, stirring to combine. Let the mixture simmer for an additional 5 minutes, allowing the flavors to meld together.
- Finish the Dish: Slice the cooked chicken breasts into strips and add them to the skillet with the lentils. Stir to combine. Add the olives, lemon juice, and lemon zest, and cook for 1-2 minutes.
- Serve: Divide the lentil and chicken mixture among four plates. Sprinkle with chopped parsley and serve hot.

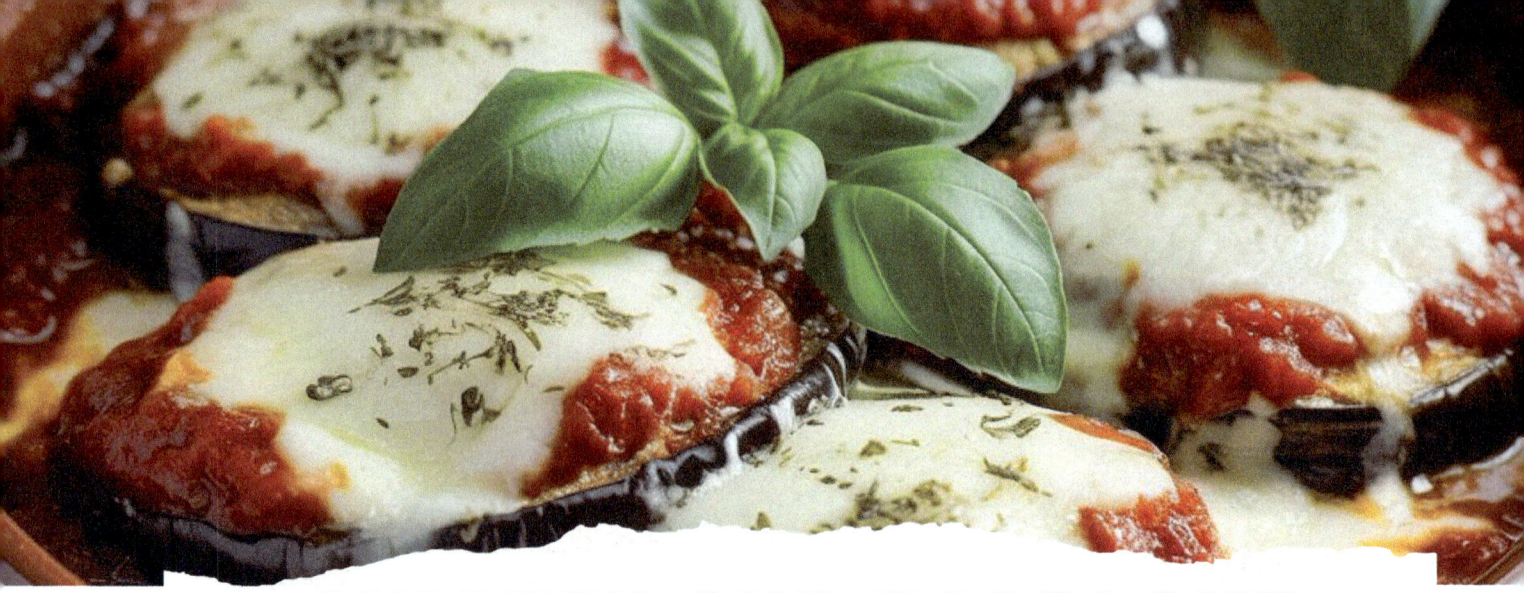

CHICKEN AND EGGPLANT BAKE

Servings: 4　　**Total Time:** 45 Min

Calories: 320 | **Protein:** 35g | **Carbohydrates:** 18g | **Fat:** 14g

Ingredients

- 4 boneless, skinless chicken breasts
- 2 medium eggplants, sliced into 1/2-inch rounds
- 1 tablespoon olive oil
- 1 teaspoon dried oregano
- 1 teaspoon garlic powder
- 1 teaspoon paprika
- Salt and pepper to taste
- 1 cup marinara sauce (preferably low-sugar)
- 1/2 cup shredded mozzarella cheese
- 1/4 cup grated Parmesan cheese
- Fresh basil for garnish

Tips

- For extra flavor, add a pinch of red pepper flakes to the marinara sauce for a bit of heat.
- You can substitute the chicken breasts for boneless, skinless chicken thighs for a juicier option.
- If you prefer a lower-fat version, use part-skim mozzarella cheese or omit the cheese entirely for a lighter dish.
- Leftovers can be stored in an airtight container in the fridge for up to 3 days. Reheat in the oven for best results.

Directions

- Preheat the oven to 375°F (190°C).
- In a large skillet, heat 1 tablespoon of olive oil over medium heat. Season the chicken breasts with oregano, garlic powder, paprika, salt, and pepper. Cook the chicken for 4-5 minutes on each side until golden brown. Remove from the skillet and set aside.
- In the same skillet, add a little more olive oil if needed, then add the eggplant slices. Cook the eggplant in batches for 2-3 minutes per side until lightly browned. Set aside.
- In a baking dish, layer the eggplant slices on the bottom. Place the cooked chicken breasts on top of the eggplant. Pour marinara sauce over the chicken and eggplant.
- Sprinkle mozzarella and Parmesan cheese evenly over the top. Bake in the oven for 20-25 minutes, or until the chicken reaches an internal temperature of 165°F (75°C) and the cheese is melted and bubbly.
- Garnish with fresh basil before serving, if desired.

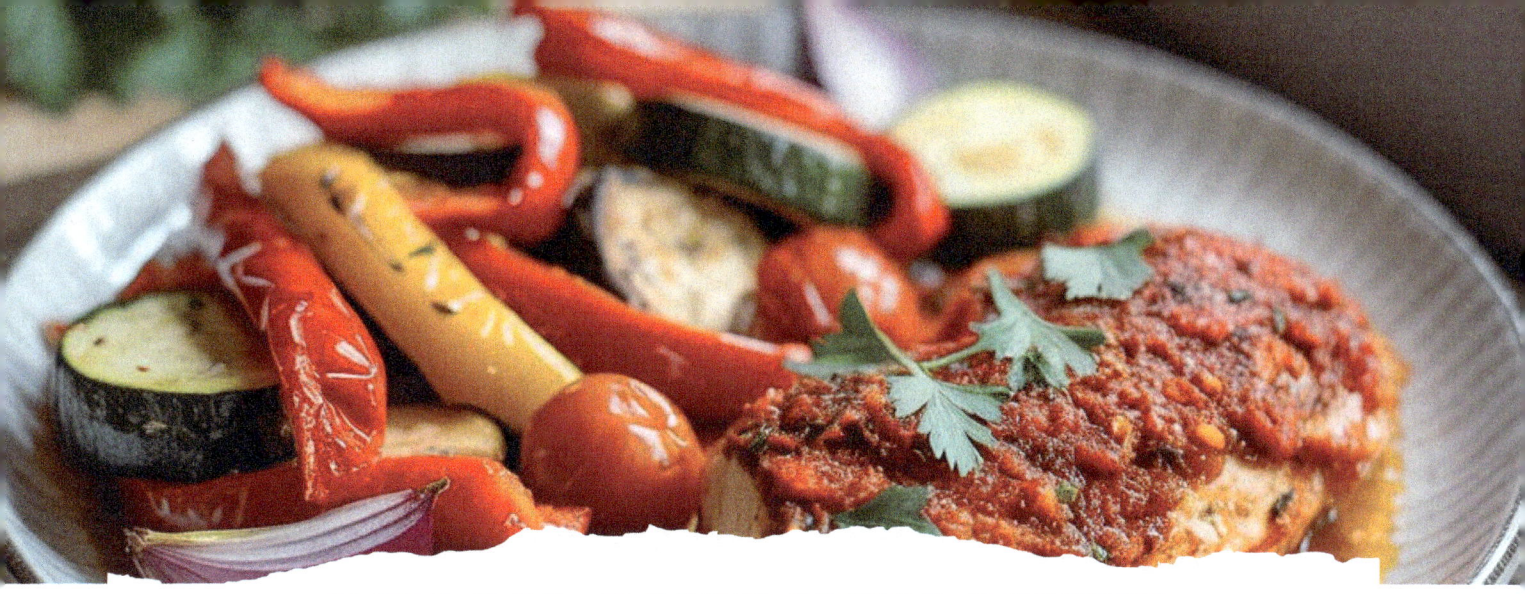

SPICY CHICKEN WITH ROASTED VEGETABLES

Servings: 2 | **Total Time:** 40 Min

Calories: 350 | **Protein:** 35g | **Carbohydrates:** 20g | **Fat:** 15g

Ingredients

- 2 boneless, skinless chicken breasts
- 1 tablespoon olive oil
- 1 teaspoon smoked paprika
- 1 teaspoon cumin
- 1/2 teaspoon cayenne pepper (adjust for spice level)
- 1/2 teaspoon garlic powder
- 1 teaspoon dried oregano
- Salt and black pepper to taste
- 1 red bell pepper, sliced
- 1 zucchini, sliced
- 1 small red onion, sliced
- 1 cup cherry tomatoes, halved
- 1 tablespoon fresh parsley, chopped (for garnish)

Directions

- Preheat your oven to 400°F (200°C).
- In a small bowl, mix together the smoked paprika, cumin, cayenne pepper, garlic powder, oregano, salt, and black pepper.
- Rub the spice mixture all over the chicken breasts, making sure to coat them evenly.
- In a large bowl, combine the sliced bell pepper, zucchini, red onion, and cherry tomatoes. Drizzle with olive oil, and toss to coat the vegetables evenly.
- Place the seasoned chicken breasts on a baking sheet lined with parchment paper. Surround the chicken with the seasoned vegetables.
- Roast in the preheated oven for 25-30 minutes, or until the chicken reaches an internal temperature of 165°F (75°C) and the vegetables are tender and slightly caramelized.
- Remove from the oven, garnish with fresh parsley, and serve hot.

Tips

- Adjust the spice level: If you prefer a milder dish, reduce or omit the cayenne pepper. For more heat, add extra cayenne or a dash of hot sauce.
- Vegetable variations: Feel free to swap the veggies for others you enjoy, such as sweet potatoes, eggplant, or broccoli.
- Meal prep: This recipe can be made ahead and stored in the fridge for up to 3 days. It also reheats beautifully for a quick lunch or dinner.

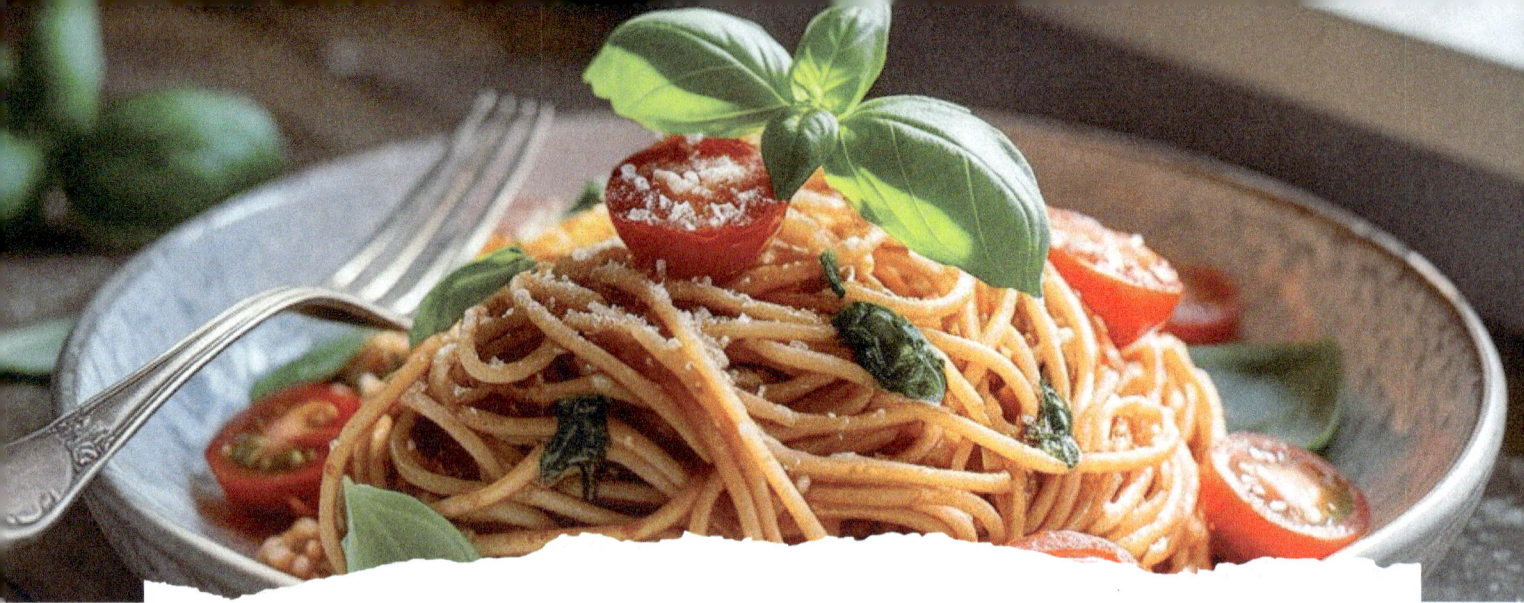

WHOLE WHEAT SPAGHETTI WITH CHERRY TOMATOES & BASIL

Servings: 2 | **Total Time:** 25 Min

Calories: 360 | **Protein:** 11g | **Carbohydrates:** 54g | **Fat:** 12g

Ingredients

- 6 oz (170g) whole wheat spaghetti
- 2 tablespoons extra-virgin olive oil
- 2 garlic cloves, minced
- 1½ cups cherry tomatoes, halved
- Salt and black pepper, to taste
- ¼ teaspoon red pepper flakes (optional)
- ½ cup fresh basil leaves, chopped
- Grated Parmesan cheese (optional, for garnish)

Directions

- Bring a large pot of salted water to a boil. Cook the whole wheat spaghetti according to package instructions until al dente. Drain and set aside, reserving ¼ cup of pasta water.
- In a large skillet, heat the olive oil over medium heat. Add the minced garlic and cook for about 1 minute, until fragrant.
- Add the cherry tomatoes to the skillet. Season with salt, pepper, and red pepper flakes if using. Sauté for 5–6 minutes, until the tomatoes soften and begin to release their juices.
- Add the cooked spaghetti to the skillet, tossing to coat. If the mixture is too dry, add a splash of the reserved pasta water.
- Stir in fresh basil and remove from heat.
- Serve warm, topped with grated Parmesan if desired.

Tips

- For extra flavor, add a splash of balsamic vinegar to the cherry tomatoes while sautéing.
- Swap basil for fresh arugula or parsley if desired.
- Add grilled chicken or shrimp for a protein boost.

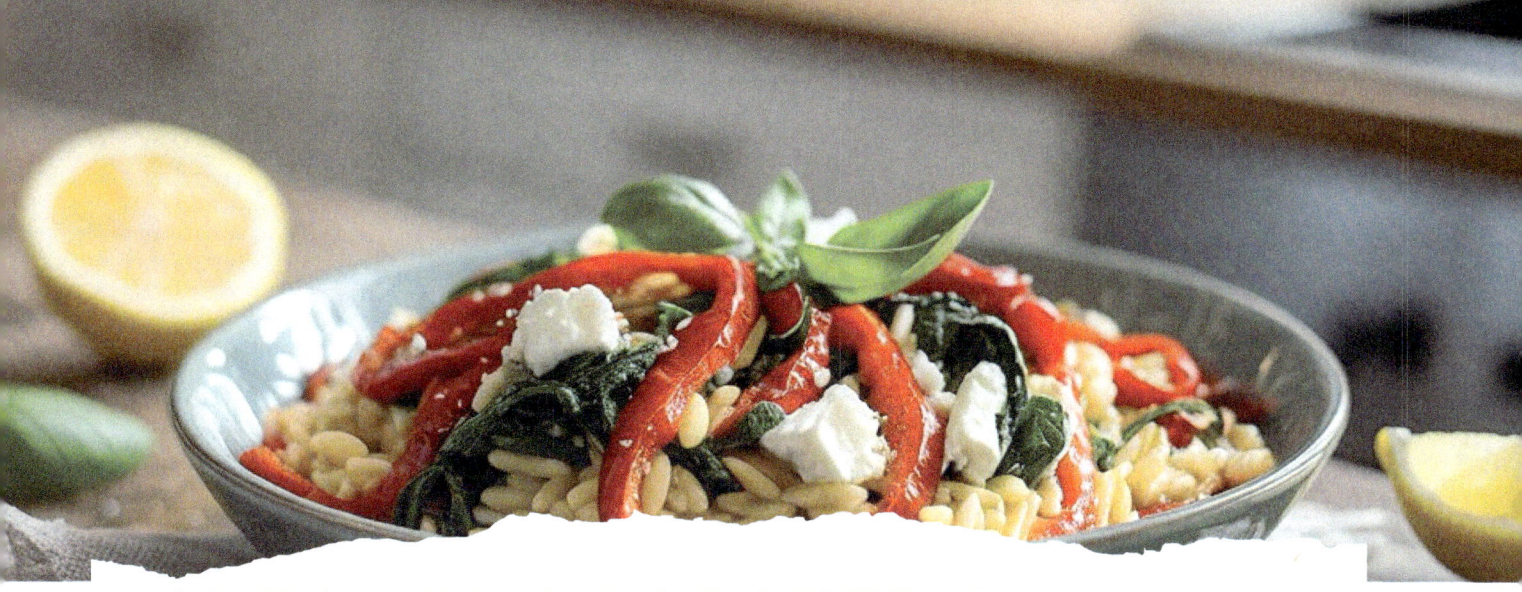

ORZO WITH ROASTED PEPPERS AND SPINACH

Servings: 4   **Total Time:** 25 Min

Calories: 260 | **Protein:** 7g | **Carbohydrates:** 35g | **Fat:** 10g

Ingredients

- 1 cup orzo pasta
- 1 tablespoon olive oil
- 2 garlic cloves, minced
- 1 cup roasted red peppers, sliced (jarred or homemade)
- 3 cups fresh spinach, chopped
- ¼ cup crumbled feta cheese
- Salt and pepper, to taste
- Juice of ½ lemon
- Fresh basil, chopped (for garnish)

Tips

- For extra flavor, add a splash of balsamic vinegar to the cherry tomatoes while sautéing.
- Swap basil for fresh arugula or parsley if desired.
- Add grilled chicken or shrimp for a protein boost.

Directions

- Bring a medium pot of salted water to a boil. Add orzo and cook according to package instructions (usually about 8–10 minutes), then drain and set aside.
- In a large skillet, heat olive oil over medium heat. Add minced garlic and sauté for 1 minute until fragrant.
- Stir in the roasted red peppers and cook for 2–3 minutes to warm through.
- Add chopped spinach and cook until wilted, about 2 minutes.
- Reduce heat to low and add the cooked orzo to the skillet. Toss everything together until well combined.
- Season with salt, pepper, and lemon juice. Stir in feta cheese if using.
- Serve warm, garnished with fresh basil.

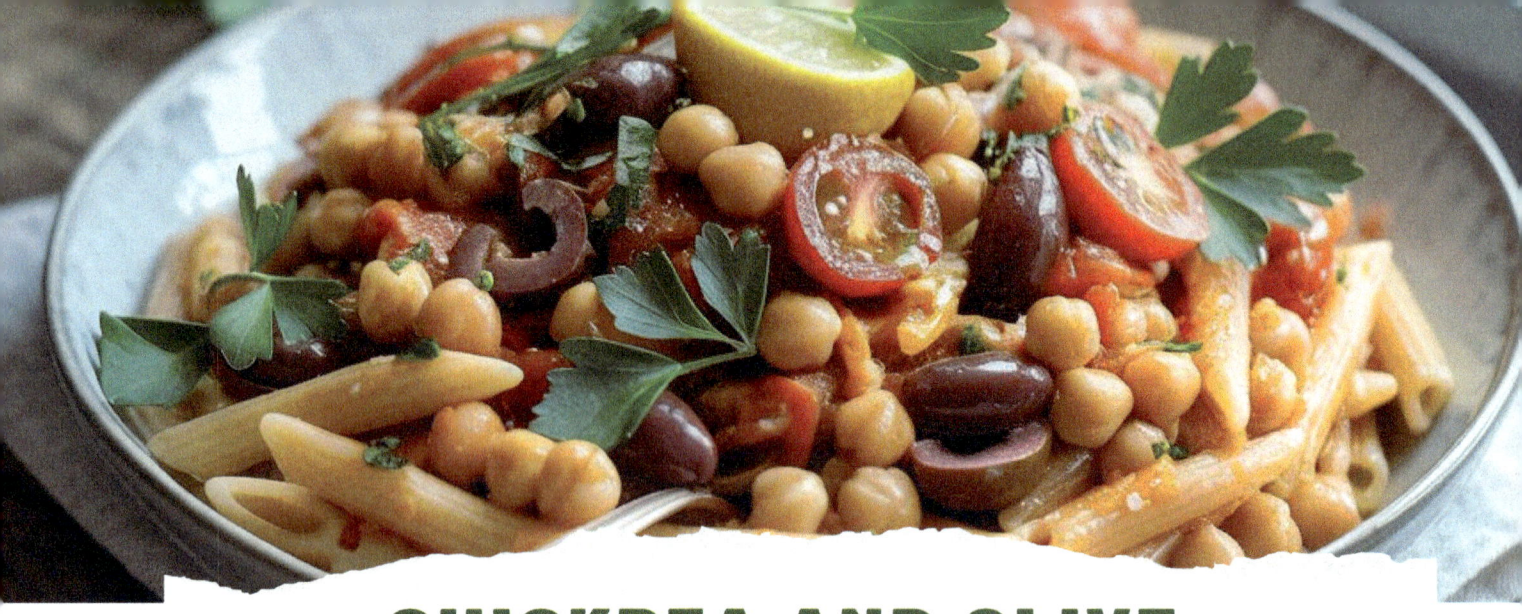

CHICKPEA AND OLIVE PASTA

Servings: 2   **Total Time:** 25 Min

Calories: 430 | **Protein:** 16g | **Carbohydrates:** 58g | **Fat:** 14g

Ingredients

- 6 oz (170g) whole wheat pasta (penne or spaghetti)
- 1 tbsp extra-virgin olive oil
- 2 cloves garlic, minced
- 1 can (15 oz) chickpeas, drained and rinsed
- 1/3 cup black or Kalamata olives, pitted and sliced
- 1/2 tsp dried oregano
- 1/4 tsp red pepper flakes
- 1 cup cherry tomatoes, halved
- Salt and black pepper to taste
- 2 tbsp chopped fresh parsley
- Juice of 1/2 lemon

Directions

- Bring a pot of salted water to a boil. Cook pasta according to package instructions until al dente. Reserve 1/4 cup of pasta water, then drain.
- In a large skillet, heat olive oil over medium heat. Add minced garlic and cook for 1 minute, until fragrant.
- Add chickpeas, olives, oregano, and red pepper flakes. Cook for 3–4 minutes, stirring often.
- Add cherry tomatoes and a splash of the reserved pasta water. Cook until tomatoes soften slightly (about 3 minutes).
- Add the cooked pasta to the skillet. Toss everything together, then season with salt, black pepper, and lemon juice.
- Sprinkle with chopped parsley and serve warm.

Tips

- Use canned low-sodium chickpeas for better heart health.
- Add a handful of spinach or arugula at the end for extra greens.
- If you're short on time, use pre-sliced olives and cherry tomatoes.
- Store leftovers in the fridge for up to 2 days – it's great cold too!

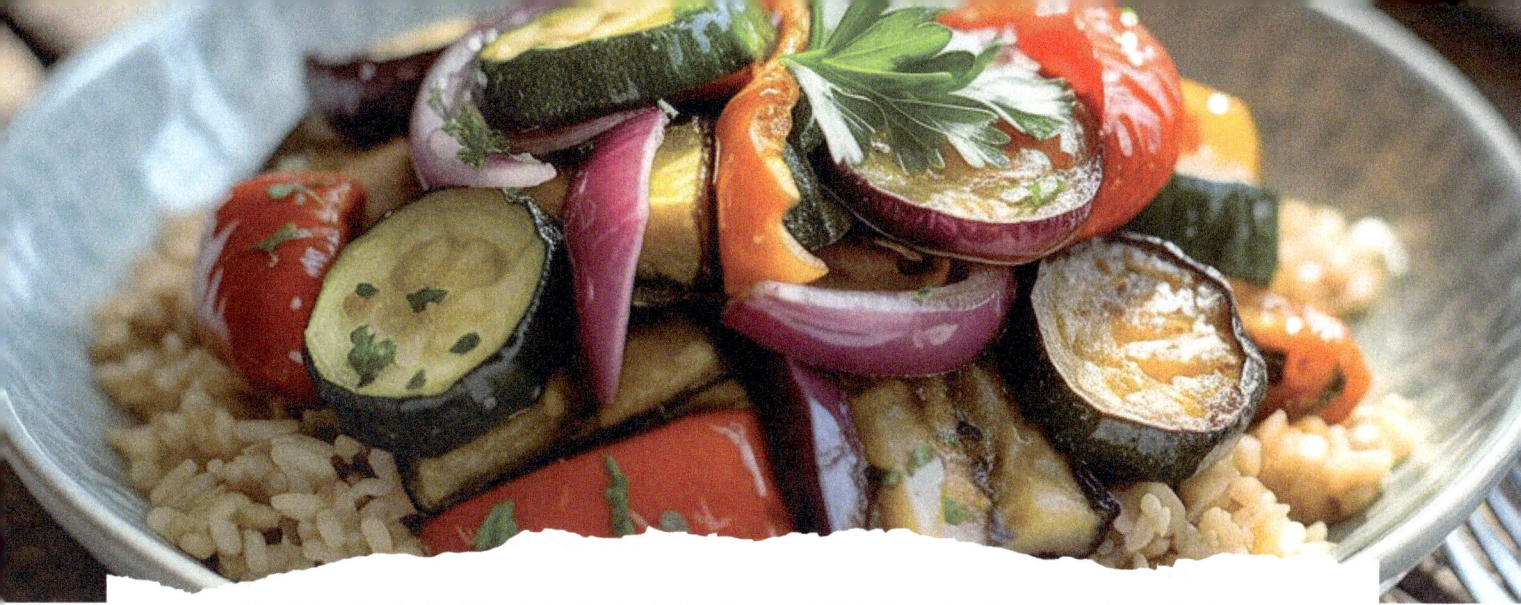

BROWN RICE WITH GRILLED VEGETABLES

Servings: 2   **Total Time:** 35 Min

Calories: 320 | **Protein:** 6g | **Carbohydrates:** 45g | **Fat:** 12g

Ingredients

- 1 cup cooked brown rice
- 1 small zucchini, sliced
- 1 red bell pepper, sliced
- 1 small eggplant, cubed
- 1 red onion, sliced
- 2 tablespoons extra-virgin olive oil
- 1 teaspoon dried oregano
- 1 teaspoon garlic powder
- Salt and pepper to taste
- 1 tablespoon lemon juice
- Fresh parsley for garnish

Directions

- Cook the brown rice according to package instructions if not already prepared. Set aside.
- Preheat your grill or grill pan over medium-high heat.
- In a large bowl, toss the zucchini, bell pepper, eggplant, and onion with olive oil, oregano, garlic powder, salt, and pepper.
- Grill the vegetables for 3–4 minutes per side, or until tender and nicely charred.
- In a large mixing bowl, combine the cooked brown rice with the grilled vegetables.
- Drizzle with lemon juice and toss gently to combine.
- Garnish with chopped fresh parsley if desired, and serve warm or at room temperature.

Tips

- For added protein, top with grilled chicken or chickpeas.
- You can use leftover rice for convenience.
- Add feta cheese crumbles for extra flavor if desired.
- Swap vegetables based on what's in season or available in your fridge.

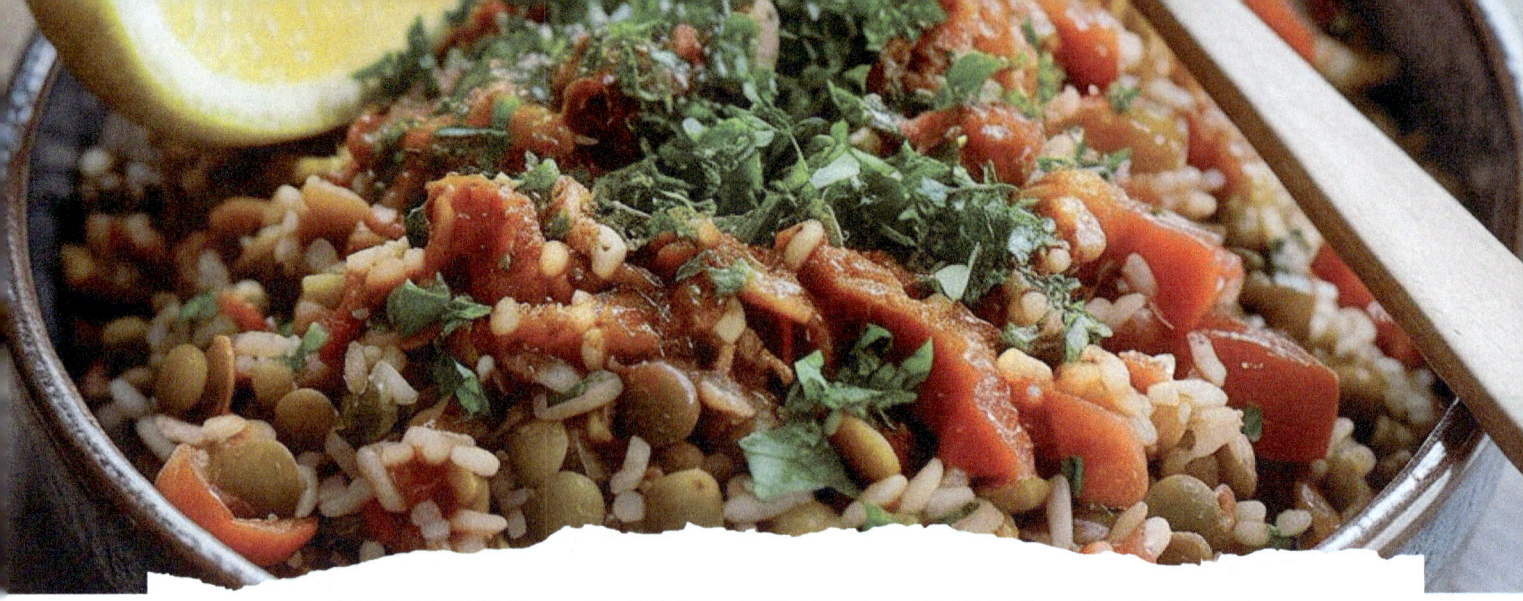

LENTIL AND TOMATO RICE BOWL

Servings: 2   **Total Time:** 35 Min

Calories: 340 | **Protein:** 13g | **Carbohydrates:** 55g | **Fat:** 7g

Ingredients

- ½ cup dry brown or green lentils, rinsed
- ¾ cup brown rice
- 1 ½ cups low-sodium vegetable broth (or water)
- 1 tablespoon extra-virgin olive oil
- 1 small onion, diced
- 2 garlic cloves, minced
- 1 cup canned diced tomatoes (no salt added)
- ½ teaspoon ground cumin
- ½ teaspoon smoked paprika
- Salt and pepper to taste
- Fresh parsley, chopped (for garnish)
- Optional: a squeeze of fresh lemon juice

Directions

- In a medium saucepan, bring lentils and 1 ½ cups water to a boil. Reduce heat and simmer for about 20–25 minutes, or until tender but not mushy. Drain any excess water.
- While the lentils cook, prepare the brown rice in a separate pot using the vegetable broth for added flavor. Simmer until fluffy (follow package instructions, typically 25–30 minutes).
- In a skillet, heat olive oil over medium heat. Add diced onion and sauté for 4–5 minutes until softened.
- Add minced garlic and cook for 1 more minute.
- Stir in diced tomatoes, cumin, paprika, salt, and pepper. Simmer for 5 minutes to let flavors meld.
- Add the cooked lentils to the tomato mixture and stir to combine. Cook for 2 more minutes.
- Divide cooked rice into bowls, top with the lentil-tomato mixture, and garnish with fresh parsley and a squeeze of lemon if desired.

Tips

- Use pre-cooked lentils and rice to save time.
- Add baby spinach or kale for extra greens.
- Store leftovers in an airtight container for up to 3 days.
- For added creaminess, top with a dollop of Greek yogurt.

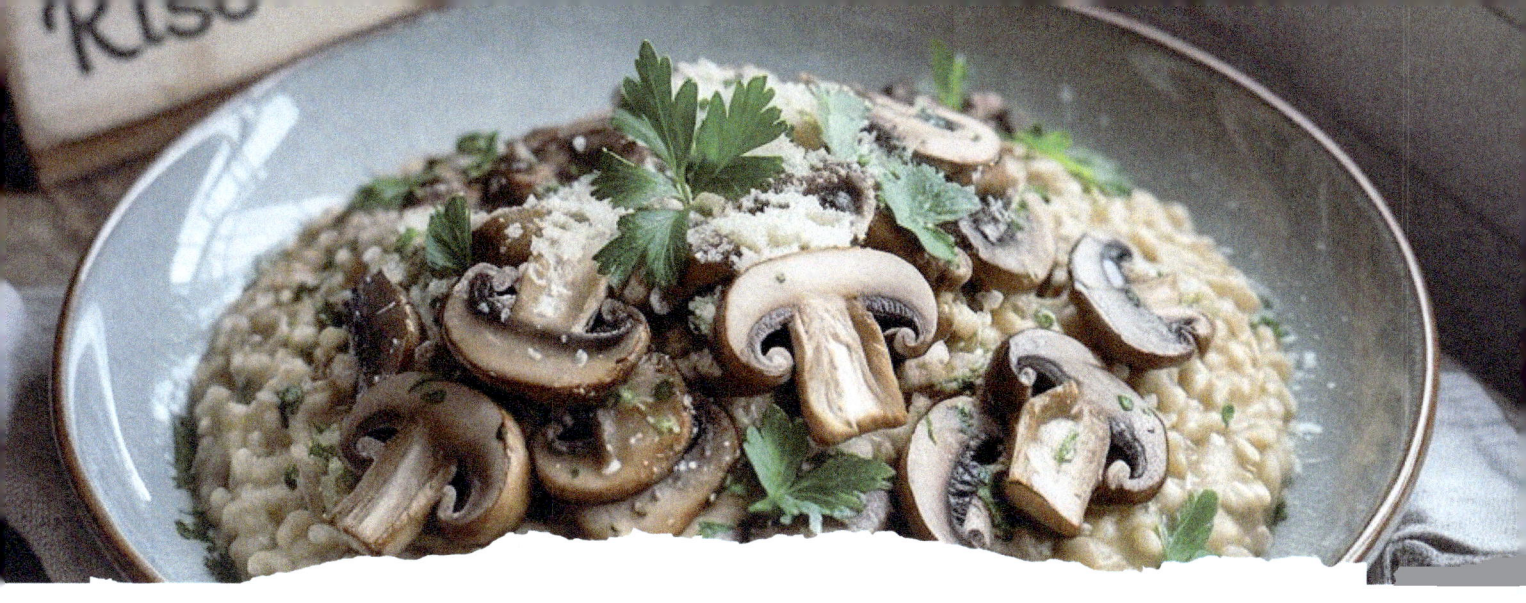

BARLEY RISOTTO WITH MUSHROOMS

Servings: 4 **Total Time:** 45 Min

Calories: 280 | **Protein:** 7g | **Carbohydrates:** 45g | **Fat:** 7g

Ingredients

- 1 tablespoon extra-virgin olive oil
- 1 small onion, finely chopped
- 2 cloves garlic, minced
- 1 cup pearl barley
- 1/2 cup dry white wine (optional – can substitute with vegetable broth)
- 4 cups low-sodium vegetable broth, warmed
- 1 cup cremini or button mushrooms, sliced
- 1/4 cup grated Parmesan cheese (optional for added creaminess)
- Salt and black pepper to taste
- 2 tablespoons chopped fresh parsley (for garnish)

Directions

- In a large pan, heat olive oil over medium heat. Sauté the chopped onion for 3–4 minutes until soft and translucent.
- Add garlic and mushrooms. Cook for another 5–6 minutes until mushrooms are browned and fragrant.
- Stir in the barley and toast for 2 minutes, allowing it to absorb the flavors.
- Pour in the wine (if using) and stir until it's mostly absorbed.
- Add the warm vegetable broth 1 cup at a time, stirring frequently and allowing each addition to absorb before adding more. This process should take about 30 minutes.
- Once the barley is tender and the mixture is creamy, stir in the Parmesan cheese (if using).
- Season with salt and black pepper to taste.
- Garnish with fresh parsley and serve warm.

Tips

- For extra protein, add white beans or shredded rotisserie chicken at the end.
- Make it dairy-free by omitting Parmesan or using a plant-based alternative.
- Stir in a handful of spinach or kale in the last few minutes for added greens.
- Use a mix of wild mushrooms for deeper flavor and texture.

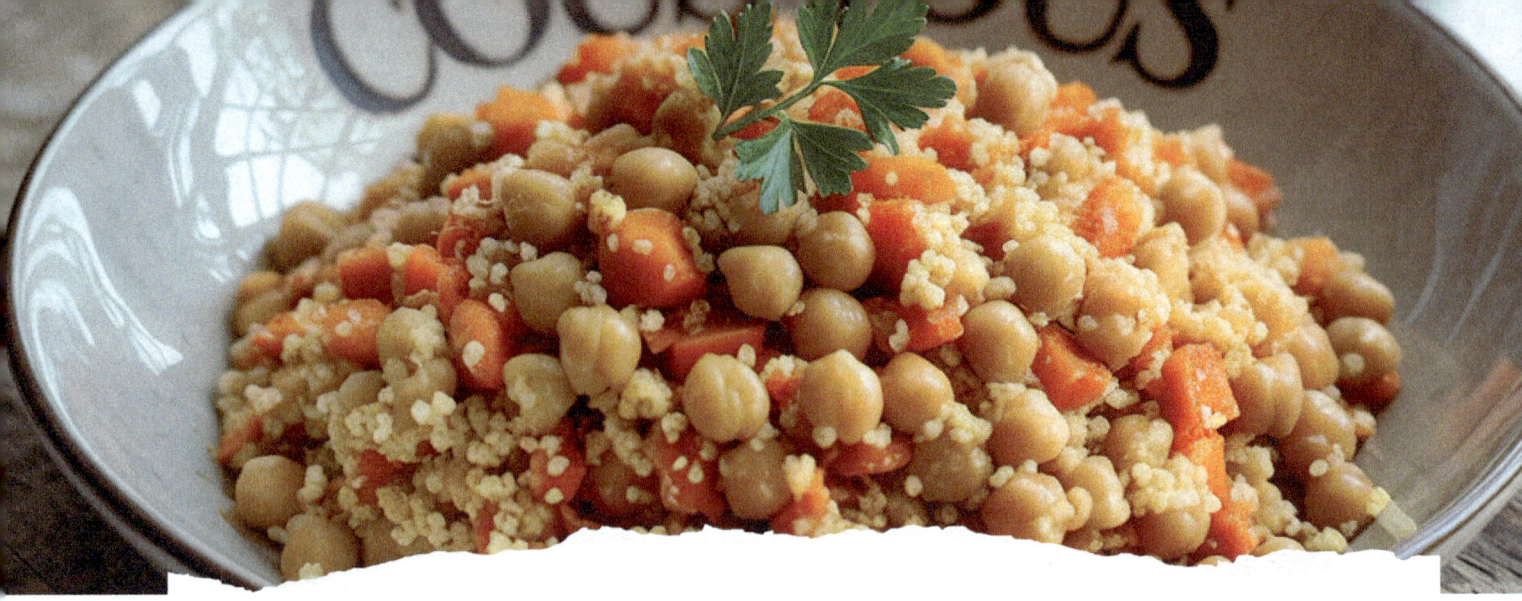

COUSCOUS WITH CHICKPEAS AND CARROTS

Servings: 4   **Total Time:** 25 Min

Calories: 310 | **Protein:** 8g | **Carbs:** 46g | **Fat:** 10g

Ingredients

- 1 cup couscous
- 1 can (15 oz) chickpeas, drained and rinsed
- 2 large carrots, peeled and sliced
- 1 tablespoon olive oil
- 1 teaspoon ground cumin
- 1 teaspoon ground coriander
- 1/2 teaspoon ground cinnamon
- Salt and pepper to taste
- 2 cups vegetable broth (or water)
- 1 tablespoon fresh parsley, chopped
- 1 tablespoon lemon juice
- 1/4 cup sliced almonds (optional)

Directions

- In a large saucepan, heat the olive oil over medium heat. Add the carrots and sauté for 5 minutes, or until slightly softened.
- Add the chickpeas, cumin, coriander, and cinnamon to the pan. Stir well to coat the vegetables and chickpeas with the spices. Cook for another 3-4 minutes, stirring occasionally.
- Pour in the vegetable broth (or water), and bring the mixture to a simmer. Once simmering, stir in the couscous. Remove from heat, cover the pan, and let it sit for about 5 minutes, or until the couscous has absorbed all the liquid.
- Fluff the couscous with a fork and stir in the lemon juice and fresh parsley. Season with salt and pepper to taste.
- Garnish with sliced almonds, if desired, and serve warm.

Tips

- For a heartier meal, add some grilled chicken or feta cheese on top.
- You can use whole wheat couscous for added fiber and a more nutty flavor.
- Make it vegan-friendly by skipping the optional feta or adding a few extra vegetables like bell peppers or zucchini.
- This dish can be served cold as a refreshing salad the next day. Simply refrigerate and enjoy!

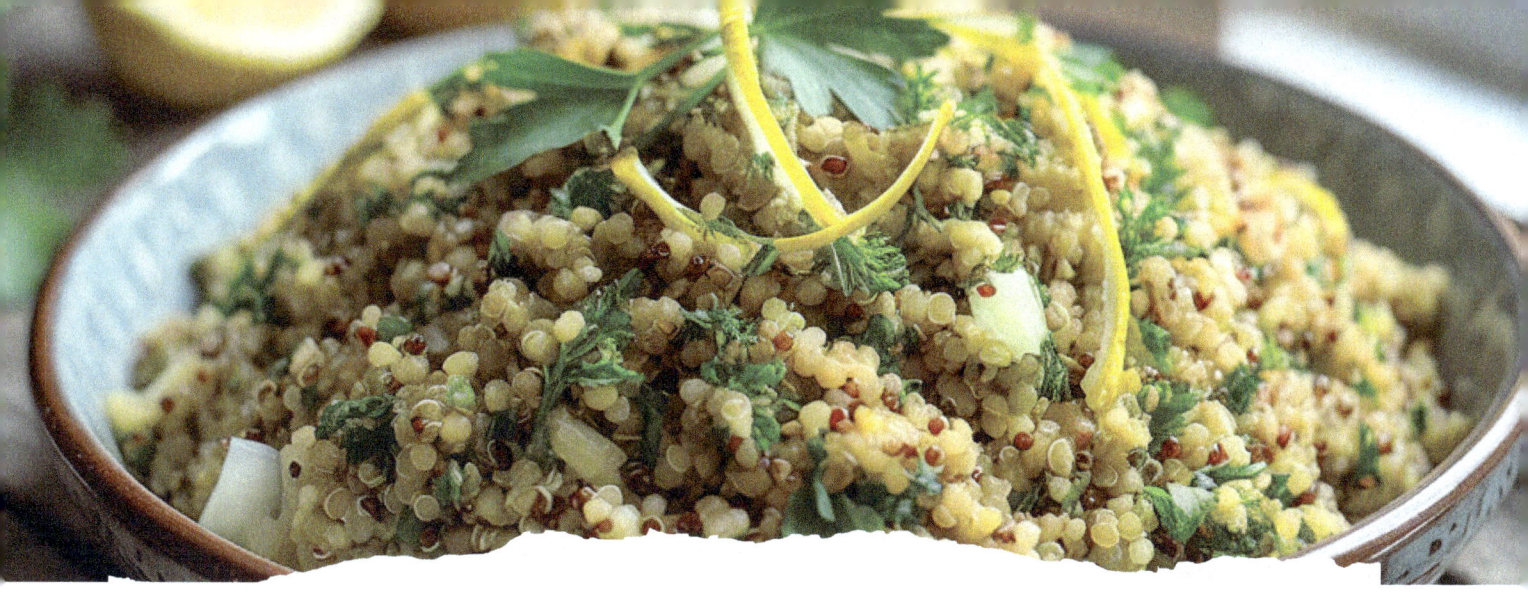

QUINOA AND LEMON PILAF

Servings: 4   **Total Time:** 30 Min

Calories: 180 | **Carbs:** 34g | **Protein:** 6g | **Fat:** 4g

Ingredients

- 1 cup quinoa, rinsed
- 2 cups vegetable broth (or water)
- 1 tablespoon olive oil
- 1 small onion, finely chopped
- 2 garlic cloves, minced
- 1/2 teaspoon ground cumin
- Zest of 1 lemon
- Juice of 1 lemon
- Salt and pepper to taste
- Fresh parsley, chopped (for garnish)

Tips

- For added flavor, you can substitute vegetable broth with chicken broth for a richer taste.
- Make it a meal by adding sautéed vegetables like zucchini or bell peppers, or even grilled chicken or shrimp for a protein boost.
- Storage: Leftovers can be stored in an airtight container in the fridge for up to 3 days. Reheat in the microwave with a splash of water or broth to restore moisture.
- Vegan-friendly: This dish is naturally vegan, making it an excellent option for plant-based meals.

Directions

- In a medium-sized pot, bring the vegetable broth (or water) to a boil over high heat.
- Stir in the quinoa, cover, and reduce heat to low. Let it simmer for 15 minutes or until the quinoa is tender and the liquid is absorbed. Remove from heat and set aside.
- In a large pan, heat the olive oil over medium heat. Add the chopped onion and sauté for 5-7 minutes until softened and translucent.
- Add the minced garlic and cumin to the pan and sauté for another 1-2 minutes until fragrant.
- Add the cooked quinoa to the pan, stirring to combine with the onions and garlic.
- Stir in the lemon zest and lemon juice, and season with salt and pepper to taste. Continue to cook for an additional 2-3 minutes, allowing the flavors to meld together.
- Remove from heat and garnish with fresh chopped parsley before serving.

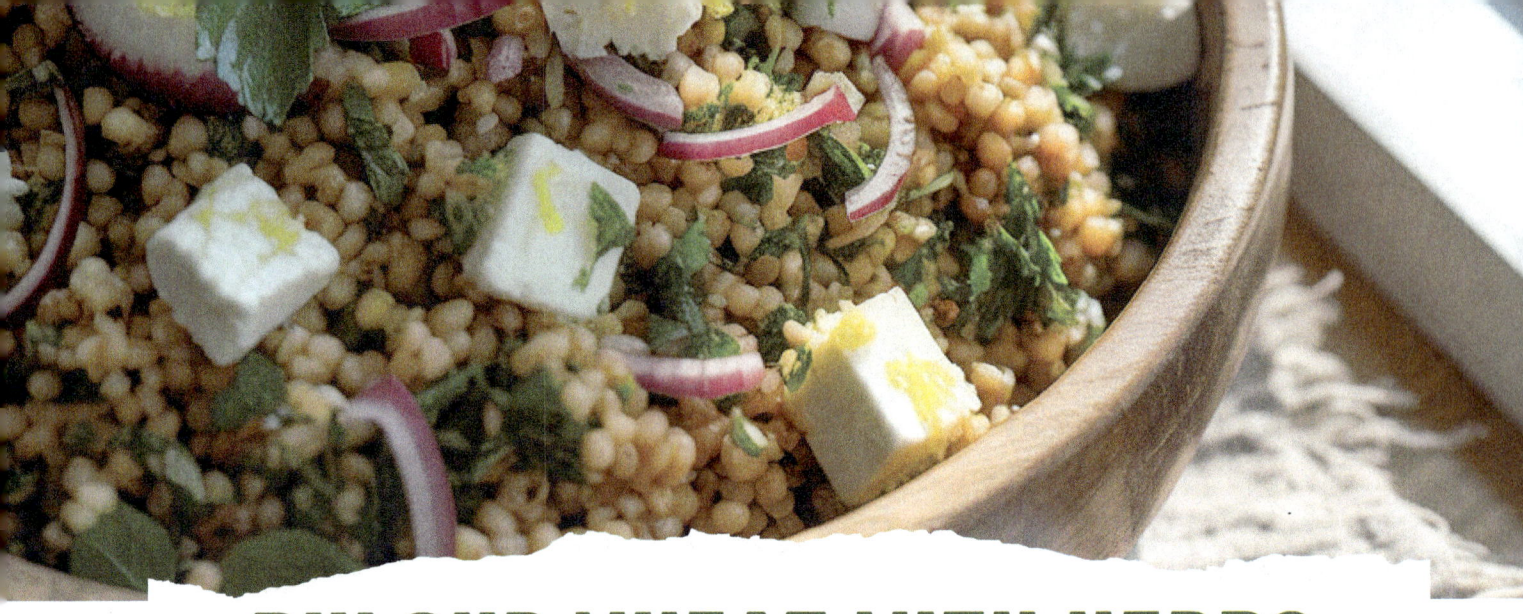

BULGUR WHEAT WITH HERBS AND FETA

Servings: 4　　**Total Time:** 25 Min

Calories: 200 | **Carbohydrates:** 30g | **Protein:** 6g | **Fat:** 8g

Ingredients

- 1 cup bulgur wheat
- 2 cups water or vegetable broth
- 1 tablespoon extra virgin olive oil
- 1 small red onion, finely chopped
- 1/2 cup fresh parsley, chopped
- 1/4 cup fresh mint, chopped
- 1/2 cup crumbled feta cheese
- 1 tablespoon lemon juice
- 1 teaspoon lemon zest
- Salt and pepper to taste

Directions

- Cook the bulgur: In a medium saucepan, bring the water or vegetable broth to a boil. Add the bulgur wheat, reduce heat to low, cover, and simmer for 12-15 minutes, or until the bulgur has absorbed all the liquid and is tender. Fluff with a fork to separate the grains.
- Prepare the herbs: While the bulgur cooks, chop the parsley, mint, and onion.
- Combine: In a large bowl, combine the cooked bulgur with the olive oil, chopped red onion, parsley, mint, and crumbled feta.
- Season: Stir in the lemon juice and zest. Season with salt and pepper to taste. Mix well to combine all the ingredients.
- Serve: Serve warm or chilled as a side dish or light meal.

Tips

- Make it a meal: For a heartier dish, add grilled chicken, lamb, or chickpeas.
- Customize the herbs: Feel free to swap in fresh basil, dill, or thyme for different flavors.
- Storage: Leftovers can be stored in an airtight container in the refrigerator for up to 3 days. The flavors even improve after a day!
- Add veggies: Roasted vegetables like zucchini or bell peppers pair wonderfully with this dish.

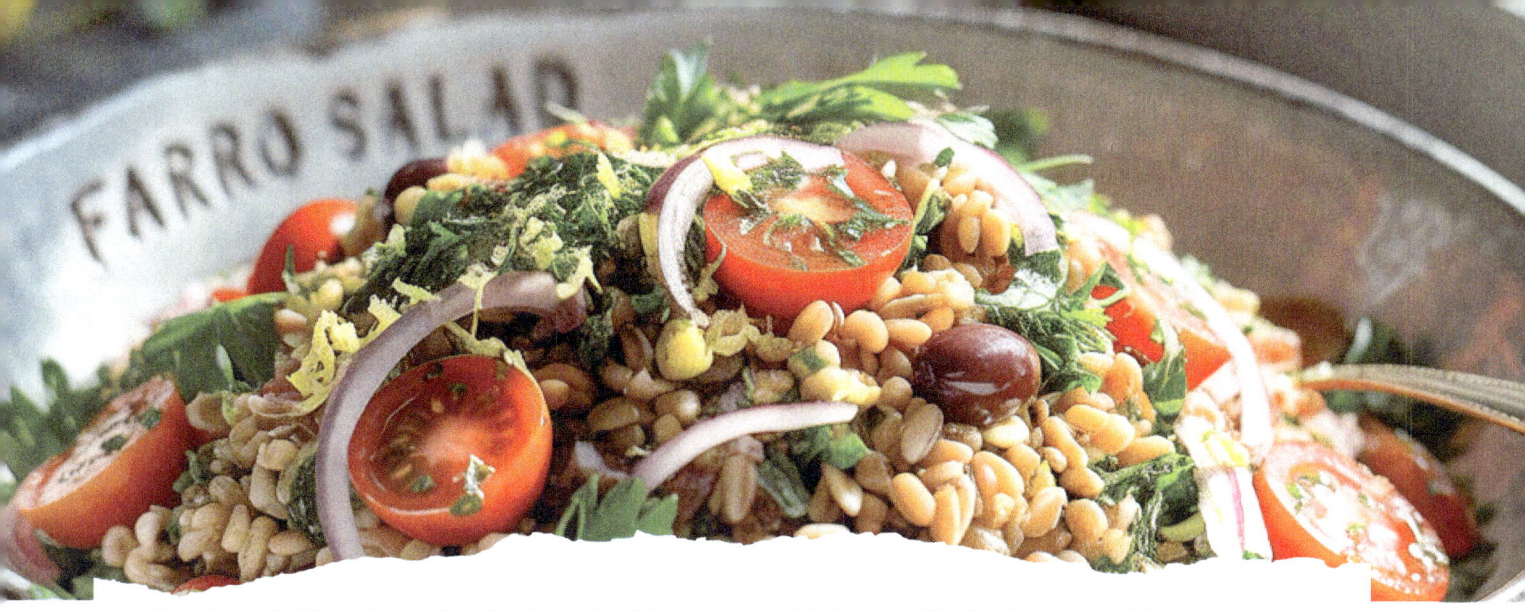

FARRO SALAD WITH TOMATOES AND OLIVES

Servings: 4 **Total Time:** 30 Min

Calories: 240 | **Protein:** 7g | **Carbohydrates:** 32g | **Fat:** 9g

Ingredients

- 1 cup farro
- 2 cups water
- 1 tablespoon extra-virgin olive oil
- 1 teaspoon lemon zest
- 1 tablespoon fresh lemon juice
- 1/2 teaspoon dried oregano
- 1/4 teaspoon salt, or to taste
- 1/4 teaspoon black pepper, or to taste
- 1 cup cherry tomatoes, halved
- 1/2 cup Kalamata olives, pitted and sliced
- 1/4 cup red onion, finely chopped
- 1/4 cup fresh parsley, chopped
- Optional: crumbled feta cheese for topping

Directions

- Cook the farro: In a medium saucepan, bring 2 cups of water to a boil. Add the farro and a pinch of salt. Lower the heat, cover, and simmer for 20-25 minutes, or until the farro is tender but still chewy. Drain any excess water and set aside to cool.
- Prepare the dressing: In a small bowl, whisk together olive oil, lemon zest, lemon juice, oregano, salt, and black pepper until well combined.
- Assemble the salad: In a large bowl, combine the cooked farro, cherry tomatoes, Kalamata olives, red onion, and parsley. Drizzle the dressing over the salad and toss gently to combine.
- Serve: If desired, sprinkle with crumbled feta cheese just before serving for an extra burst of flavor.

Tips

- For a gluten-free option, swap farro for quinoa or brown rice.
- To make this salad a more filling meal, add grilled chicken or chickpeas for extra protein.
- This salad can be made ahead and stored in the fridge for up to 2 days. The flavors will deepen as it sits.
- If you prefer a milder taste, rinse the red onion in cold water before adding it to the salad to reduce its sharpness.

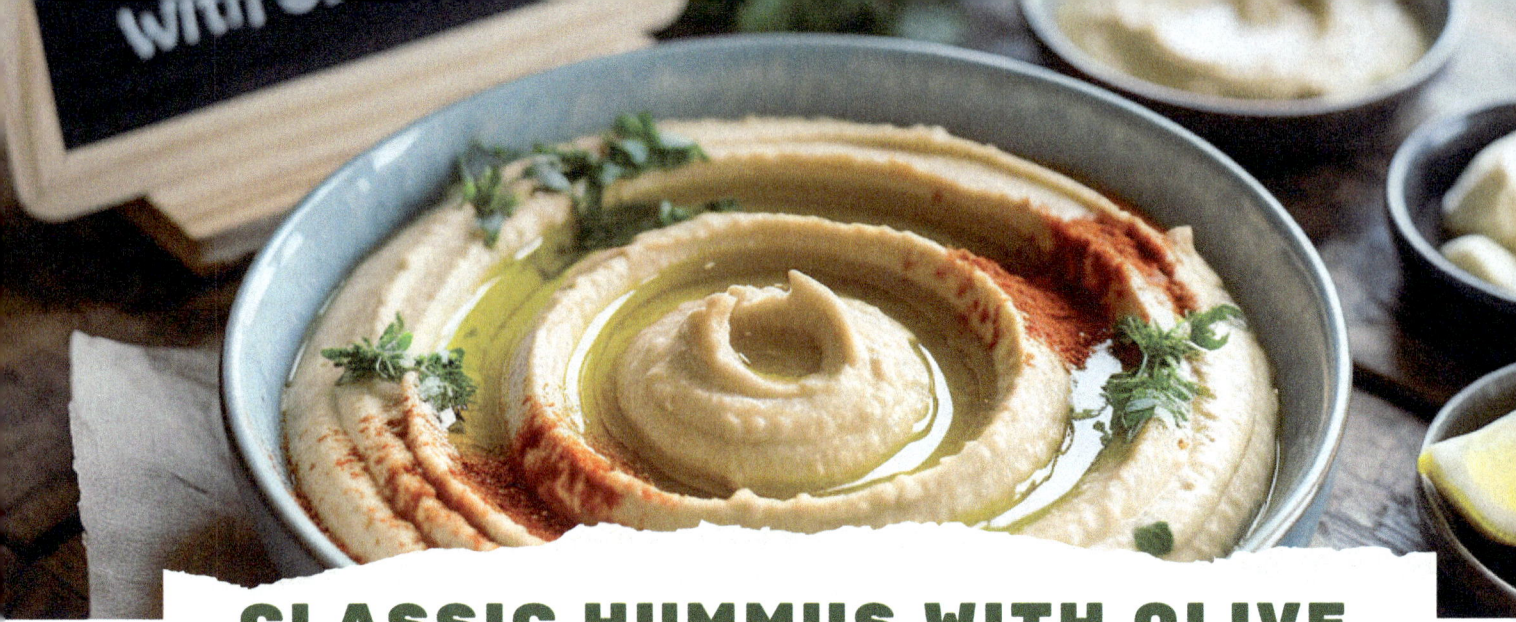

CLASSIC HUMMUS WITH OLIVE OIL

Servings: 8 **Total Time:** 10 Min

Calories: 150 | **Protein:** 4g | **Carbohydrates:** 15g | **Fat:** 9g

Ingredients

- 1 can (15 oz) of chickpeas, drained and rinsed
- 1/4 cup tahini
- 2 tablespoons extra-virgin olive oil, plus more for drizzling
- 1 garlic clove, minced
- 2 tablespoons fresh lemon juice
- 1/2 teaspoon ground cumin
- Salt, to taste
- Water, as needed for desired consistency
- Fresh parsley, chopped (for garnish)
- Paprika (optional, for garnish)

Directions

- Blend the Ingredients: In a food processor or high-powered blender, combine the chickpeas, tahini, olive oil, garlic, lemon juice, cumin, and salt. Process until smooth. If the hummus is too thick, add water one tablespoon at a time and continue blending until you reach your desired consistency.
- Taste & Adjust: Taste the hummus and adjust the seasoning, adding more salt, lemon juice, or cumin as needed.
- Serve: Transfer the hummus to a serving dish. Drizzle with extra olive oil and sprinkle with chopped parsley and paprika for a touch of color and flavor.
- Enjoy: Serve with pita bread, fresh veggies, or as a spread on sandwiches.

Tips

- For an even creamier texture, peel the skins off the chickpeas before blending. It takes a little extra time, but it makes a big difference!
- Add a bit of roasted red pepper or sun-dried tomatoes to the blend for a twist on the classic flavor.
- Store leftover hummus in an airtight container in the fridge for up to 4-5 days. It also freezes well for up to 1 month.

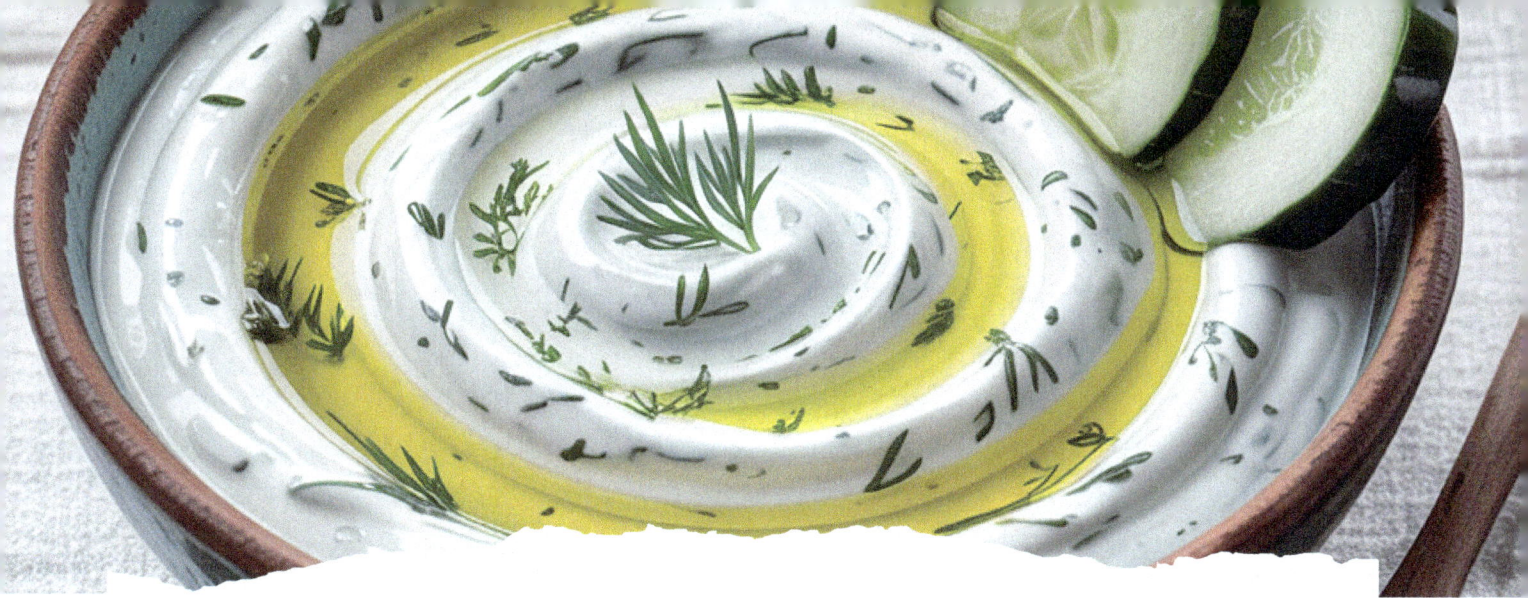

TZATZIKI CUCUMBER YOGURT DIP

Servings: 4 **Total Time:** 10 Min

Calories: 90 | **Protein:** 7g | **Carbohydrates:** 6g | **Fat:** 5g

Ingredients

- 1 cup plain Greek yogurt
- 1 cucumber, grated and excess water squeezed out
- 1 tablespoon extra virgin olive oil
- 1 tablespoon fresh lemon juice
- 1 garlic clove, minced
- 1 tablespoon fresh dill, chopped (or 1 teaspoon dried dill)
- Salt and pepper to taste

Directions

- In a medium-sized bowl, combine the Greek yogurt, grated cucumber, and olive oil.
- Add the lemon juice, minced garlic, and fresh dill to the bowl.
- Stir everything together until smooth and well incorporated.
- Season with salt and pepper to taste.
- Chill in the refrigerator for 30 minutes before serving to allow the flavors to meld together.
- Serve as a dip with pita, fresh vegetables, or as a topping for grilled meats.

Tips

- For extra creaminess: Use full-fat Greek yogurt for a richer texture.
- Make it ahead: Tzatziki is even better after sitting in the fridge for a few hours or overnight, as the flavors have more time to develop.
- Customize the flavor: Add a pinch of cumin or a small amount of chopped mint for a different twist.

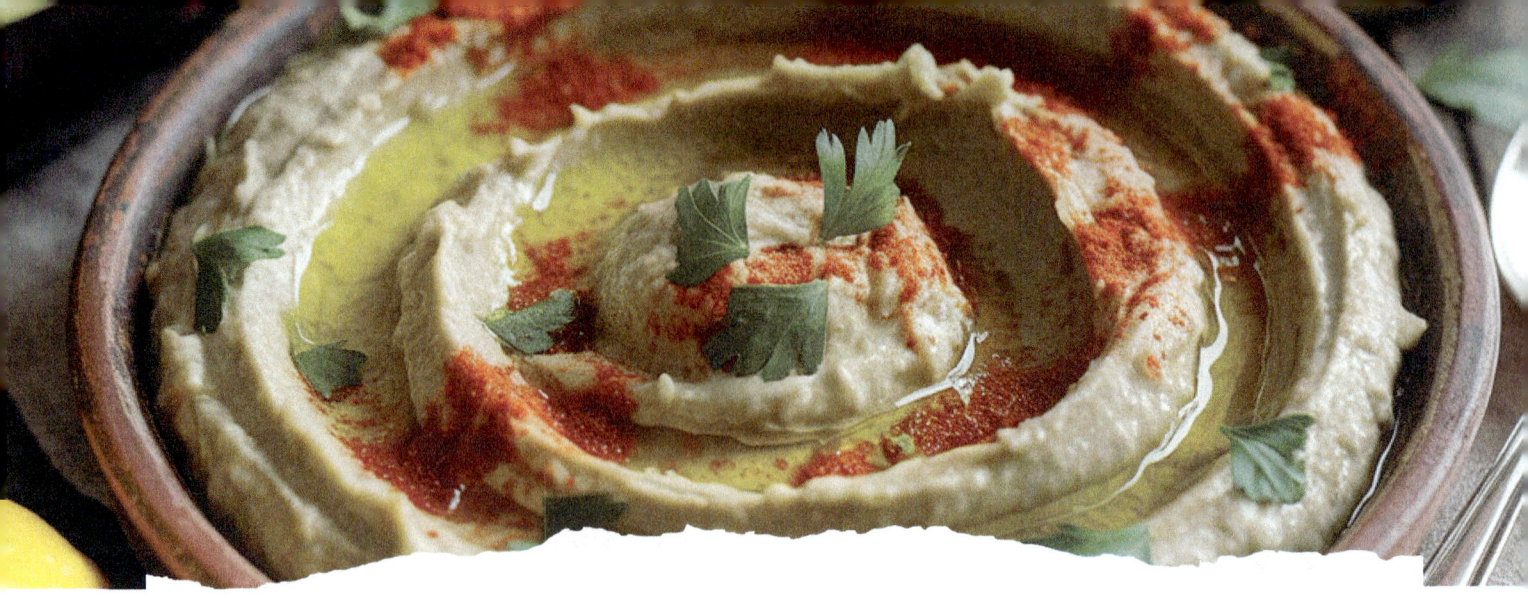

ROASTED EGGPLANT DIP (BABA GANOUSH)

Servings: 4   **Total Time:** 45 Min

Calories: 110 | **Protein:** 2g | **Carbohydrates:** 7g | **Fiber:** 3g | **Fat:** 9g

Ingredients

- 1 large eggplant
- 2 tablespoons tahini
- 2 tablespoons extra-virgin olive oil
- 1 garlic clove, minced
- Juice of 1 lemon
- Salt to taste
- 1 tablespoon chopped parsley (optional, for garnish)
- Paprika or smoked paprika (optional, for garnish)

Directions

- Preheat oven to 400°F (200°C).
- Pierce the eggplant a few times with a fork. Place on a baking sheet and roast for 35–40 minutes, until the skin is charred and the inside is soft.
- Let cool for 5–10 minutes, then cut the eggplant in half and scoop out the flesh into a bowl.
- Add tahini, olive oil, garlic, lemon juice, and salt. Mash with a fork or blend with a food processor until smooth and creamy.
- Taste and adjust seasoning, adding more lemon juice or salt if desired.
- Serve in a bowl, garnished with chopped parsley and a dash of paprika or smoked paprika.

Tips

- For a smokier flavor, grill the eggplant instead of roasting.
- Chill before serving for best taste.
- Pairs perfectly with whole grain pita, raw veggies, or as a sandwich spread.

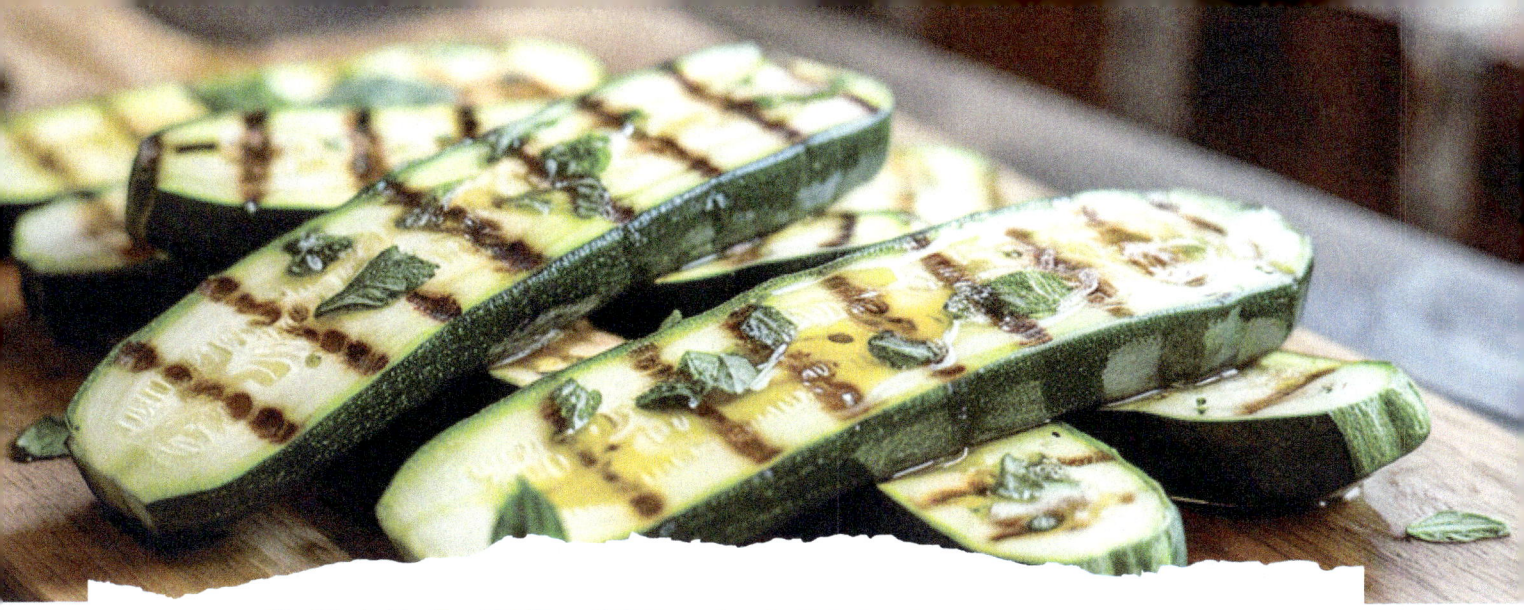

GRILLED ZUCCHINI WITH MINT

Servings: 4   **Total Time:** 20 Min

Calories: 110 | **Protein:** 2g | **Carbohydrates:** 7g | **Fiber:** 3g | **Fat:** 9g

Ingredients

- 4 medium zucchinis, sliced lengthwise
- 2 tablespoons extra-virgin olive oil
- 1 tablespoon fresh lemon juice
- Salt and black pepper, to taste
- 2 tablespoons fresh mint leaves, finely chopped
- 1 garlic clove, minced

Directions

- Preheat a grill or grill pan over medium heat.
- Brush both sides of the zucchini slices with olive oil and season with salt and pepper.
- Grill zucchini slices for 3–4 minutes on each side, until tender and lightly charred.
- Transfer grilled zucchini to a plate and drizzle with lemon juice.
- Sprinkle chopped mint and minced garlic (if using) over the top.
- Serve warm or at room temperature.

Tips

- For extra flavor, add a sprinkle of crumbled feta or a dash of balsamic glaze.
- This dish pairs wonderfully with grilled fish or whole grain couscous.
- Mint can be substituted with fresh parsley or basil for a different flavor twist.

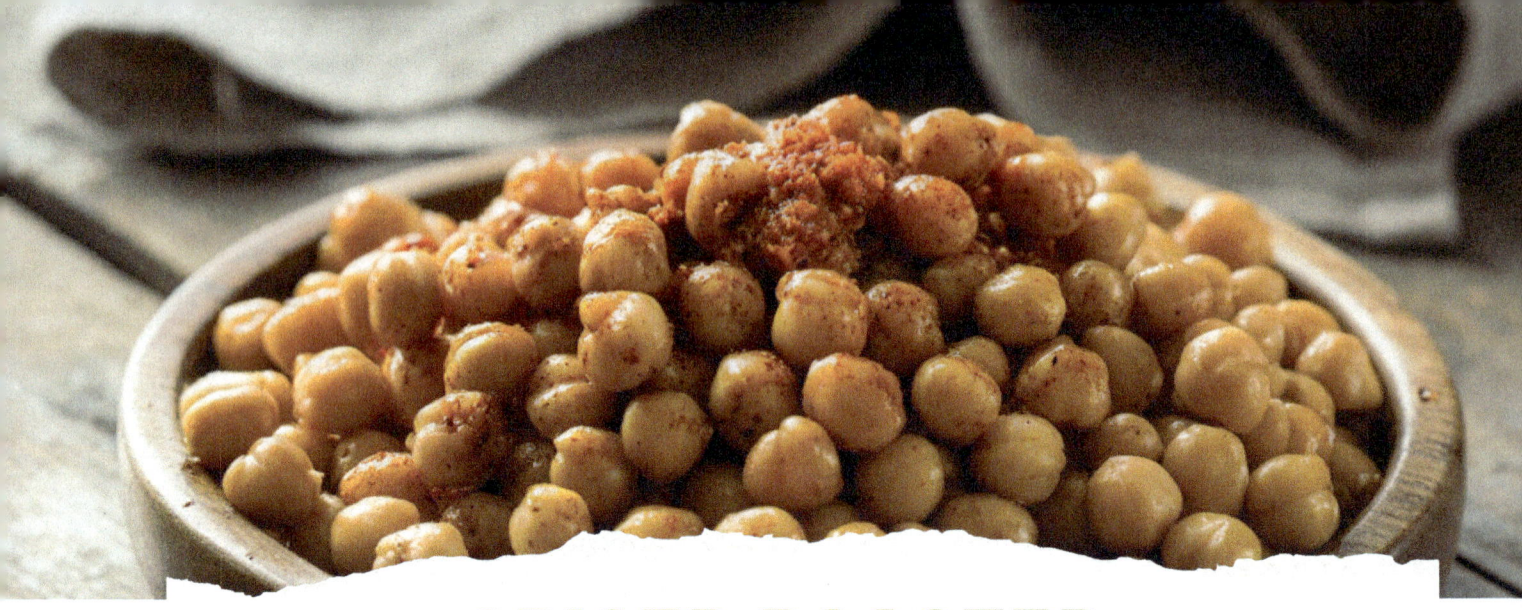

SPICED ROASTED CHICKPEAS

Servings: 4 | **Total Time:** 35 Min

Calories: 130 | **Protein:** 5g | **Carbohydrates:** 18g | **Fat:** 4.5g

Ingredients

- 1 can (15 oz) chickpeas (garbanzo beans), drained and rinsed
- 1 tablespoon olive oil
- ½ teaspoon smoked paprika
- ½ teaspoon ground cumin
- ¼ teaspoon garlic powder
- ¼ teaspoon cayenne pepper (optional, for heat)
- ¼ teaspoon salt

Directions

- Preheat oven to 400°F (200°C). Line a baking sheet with parchment paper.
- Pat chickpeas dry using a clean kitchen towel or paper towels. Removing excess moisture helps them roast evenly and turn crispy.
- Toss chickpeas in a bowl with olive oil, paprika, cumin, garlic powder, cayenne (if using), and salt until evenly coated.
- Spread chickpeas in a single layer on the prepared baking sheet.
- Roast for 25–30 minutes, shaking the pan halfway through, until golden brown and crisp.
- Cool slightly before serving. They'll continue to crisp up as they cool.

Tips

- Store leftovers in an airtight container at room temperature for up to 3 days – but they're best eaten fresh!
- Feel free to experiment with different spices like curry powder, chili lime, or Italian herbs.
- For extra crispiness, roast chickpeas for an additional 5 minutes but watch closely to prevent burning.

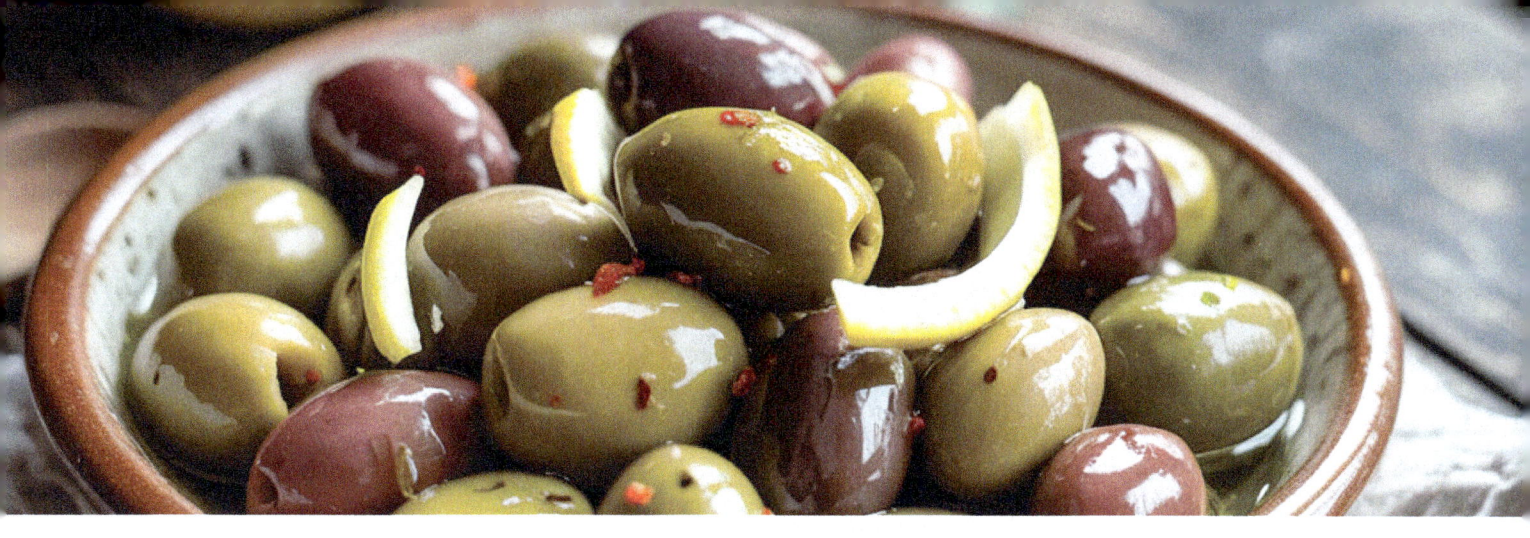

MARINATED OLIVES WITH LEMON AND GARLIC

Servings: 4   **Total Time:** 10 Min

Calories: 110 | **Fat:** 10g | **Saturated Fat**: 1.5g | **Carbohydrates:** 4g

Ingredients

- 2 cups mixed olives (green and black, pitted or whole)
- 2 tablespoons extra-virgin olive oil
- 2 cloves garlic, thinly sliced
- 1 lemon (zest and juice)
- 1 teaspoon dried oregano
- 1/2 teaspoon crushed red pepper flakes
- Fresh parsley, chopped (for garnish)

Directions

- In a medium bowl, combine olives, olive oil, sliced garlic, lemon zest, and lemon juice.
- Sprinkle in oregano and red pepper flakes if using. Toss gently to coat all the olives evenly.
- Transfer to a jar or airtight container and refrigerate for at least 2 hours, preferably overnight, to allow flavors to meld.
- Before serving, let olives come to room temperature. Garnish with fresh parsley if desired.

Tips

- Use high-quality olives for the best flavor – Kalamata, Castelvetrano, or Manzanilla work beautifully.
- Add a sprig of rosemary or a few strips of roasted red pepper for extra flavor variation.
- Keeps well in the refrigerator for up to a week – great for prepping ahead!

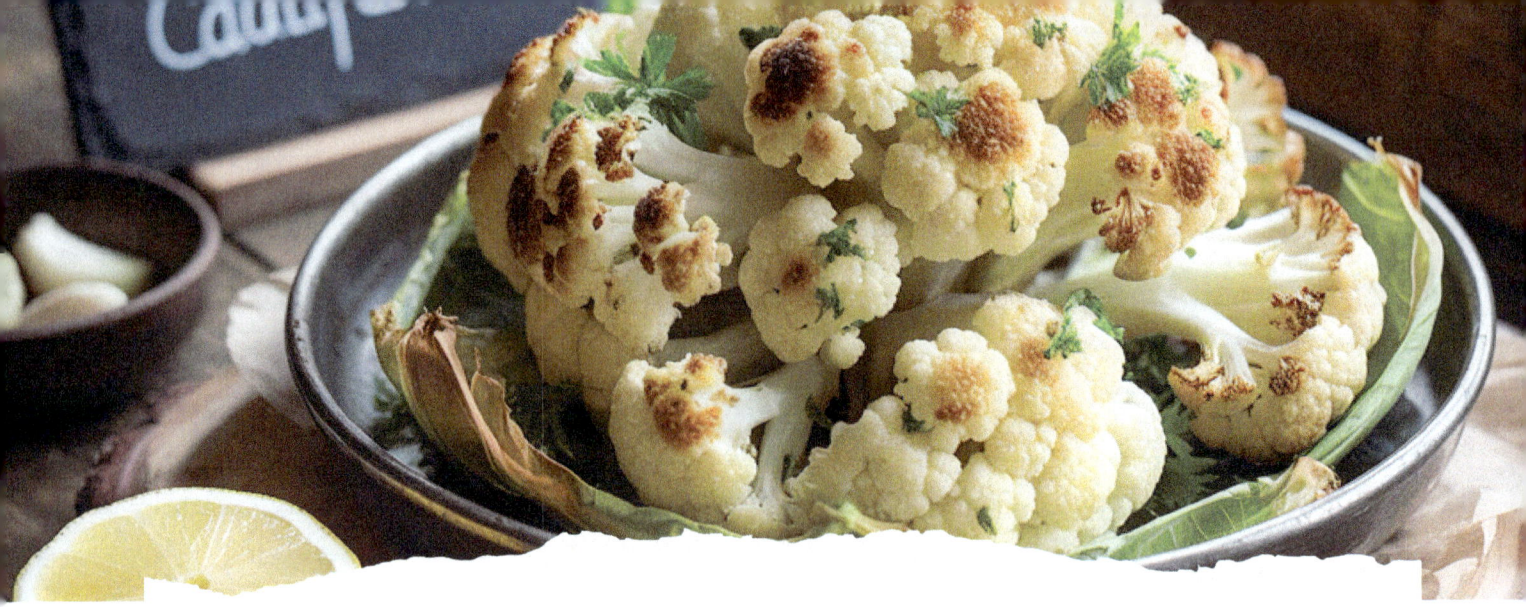

GARLIC ROASTED CAULIFLOWER

Servings: 4   **Total Time:** 30 Min

Calories: 120 | **Protein:** 3g | **Carbohydrates:** 10g | **Fat:** 9g

Ingredients

- 1 large head of cauliflower, cut into florets
- 3 tablespoons extra-virgin olive oil
- 4 garlic cloves, minced
- 1 teaspoon dried oregano
- ½ teaspoon paprika (optional for extra flavor)
- Salt and black pepper, to taste
- 2 tablespoons fresh parsley, chopped (for garnish)
- Juice of ½ lemon

Directions

- Preheat your oven to 425°F (220°C).
- In a large bowl, toss the cauliflower florets with olive oil, minced garlic, oregano, paprika (if using), salt, and pepper until evenly coated.
- Spread the cauliflower in a single layer on a baking sheet lined with parchment paper.
- Roast in the oven for 25 minutes, flipping halfway through, until the cauliflower is golden and tender with crisp edges.
- Remove from the oven, drizzle with lemon juice if desired, and sprinkle with chopped parsley before serving.

Tips

- For added crunch, sprinkle with a tablespoon of grated Parmesan cheese during the last 5 minutes of roasting.
- Make it spicy by adding a pinch of red pepper flakes.
- Pairs perfectly with grilled fish, chicken, or served as a warm side salad.

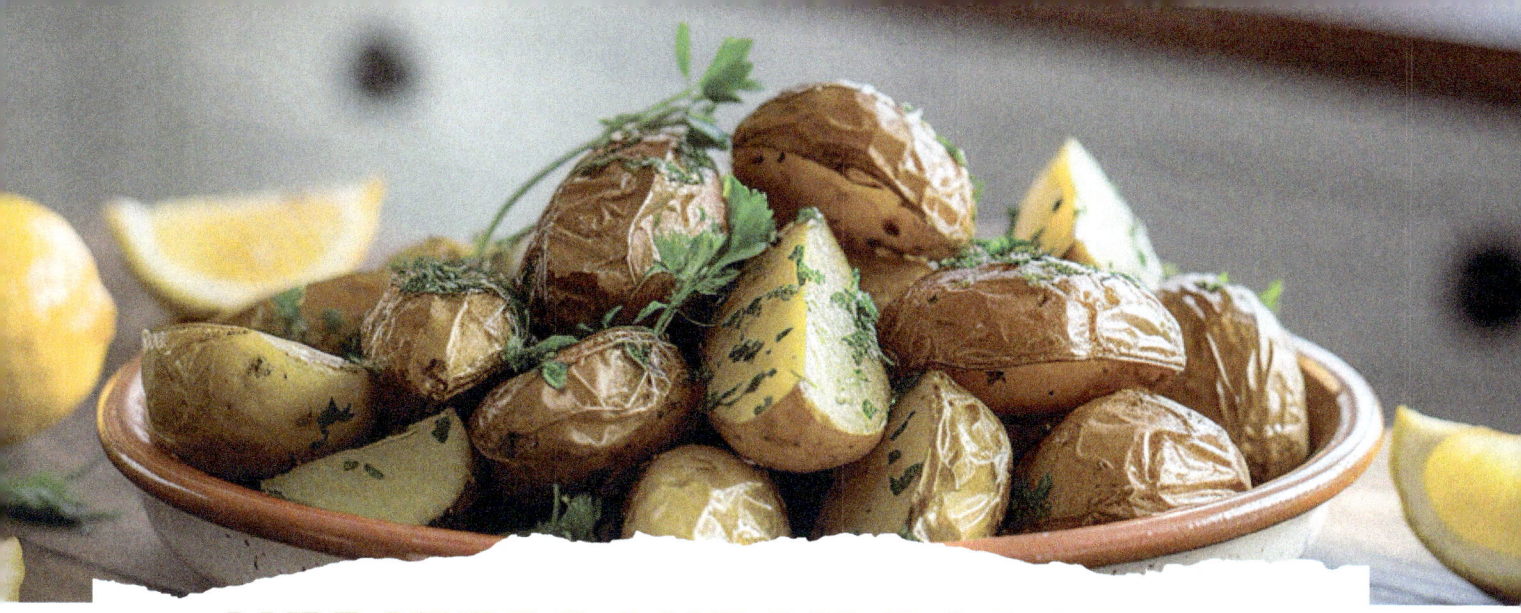

MEDITERRANEAN ROASTED POTATOES

Servings: 4 | **Total Time:** 45 Min

Calories: 210 | **Fat:** 10g | **Carbohydrates:** 27g | **Protein:** 3g

Ingredients

- 2 lbs (900g) baby potatoes, halved
- 3 tbsp extra virgin olive oil
- 1 tsp dried oregano
- 1/2 tsp dried thyme
- 1/2 tsp paprika
- 4 garlic cloves, minced
- Juice of 1 lemon
- Salt and pepper, to taste
- 2 tbsp fresh parsley, chopped (for garnish)

Directions

- Preheat your oven to 400°F (200°C).
- In a large bowl, toss the halved potatoes with olive oil, oregano, thyme, paprika, minced garlic, lemon juice, salt, and pepper until evenly coated.
- Spread the potatoes in a single layer on a baking sheet lined with parchment paper.
- Roast for 35–40 minutes, flipping halfway through, until golden brown and crispy on the edges.
- Remove from the oven, sprinkle with fresh parsley, and serve warm.

Tips

- For extra crispiness, soak the potato halves in cold water for 15 minutes, then pat dry before roasting.
- Add kalamata olives or a sprinkle of crumbled feta for extra Mediterranean flair.
- Pairs perfectly with grilled fish or a fresh Greek salad.

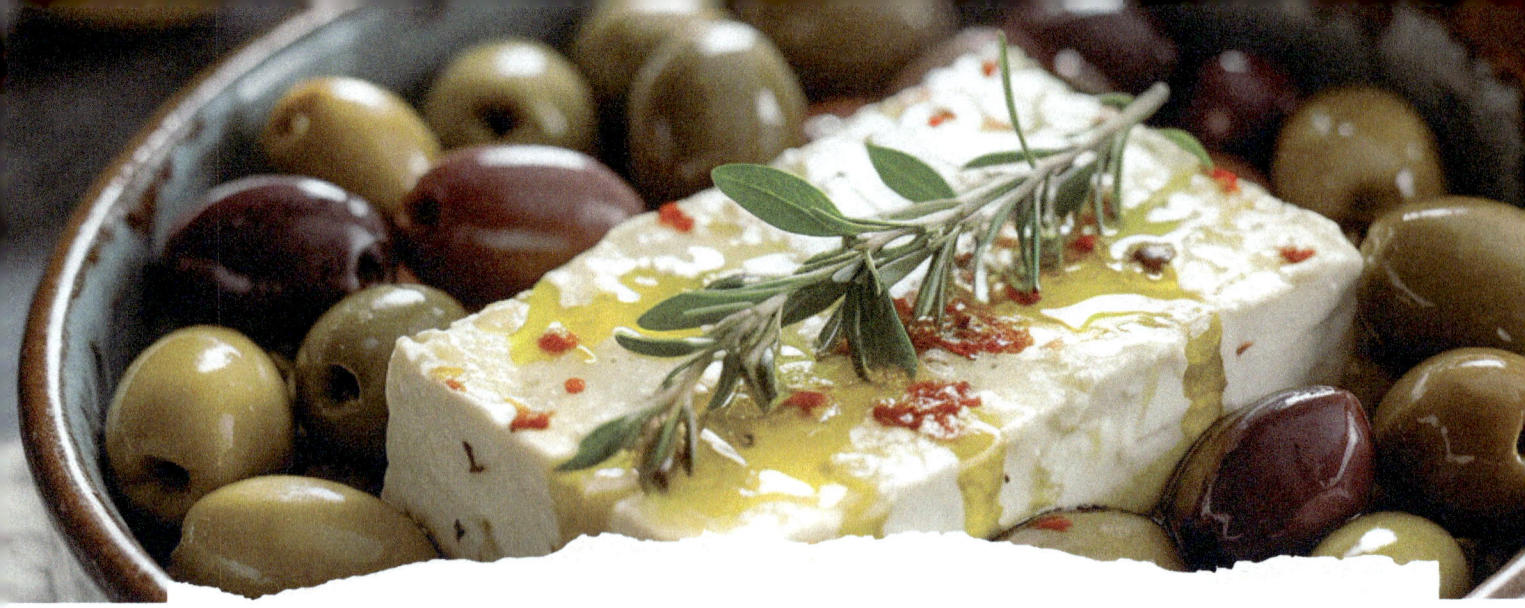

BAKED FETA AND OLIVES

Servings: 4   **Total Time:** 25 Min

Calories: 210 | **Protein:** 6g | **Fat:** 18g | **Carbohydrates:** 3g

Ingredients

- 1 block (7 oz / 200g) of feta cheese
- 1 cup mixed olives (green and black), pitted
- 2 tablespoons extra-virgin olive oil
- 1 teaspoon dried oregano
- 1/2 teaspoon red pepper flakes (optional)
- 1 clove garlic, thinly sliced
- 1 tablespoon fresh lemon juice
- Fresh parsley, chopped (for garnish)
- Crusty whole grain bread or pita (optional, for serving)

Directions

- Preheat your oven to 375°F (190°C).
- Place the block of feta in a small oven-safe dish.
- Scatter the olives around the feta.
- Drizzle olive oil evenly over the cheese and olives.
- Sprinkle with oregano, red pepper flakes, and garlic slices.
- Bake for 20 minutes, until the feta is soft and lightly golden on top.
- Remove from oven, drizzle with lemon juice, and garnish with fresh parsley.
- Serve warm with crusty bread or pita, if desired.

Tips

- Use a high-quality feta packed in brine for the best flavor and texture.
- Add cherry tomatoes to the baking dish for a juicier twist.
- This dish also pairs beautifully with grilled chicken or served over cooked quinoa for a light meal.

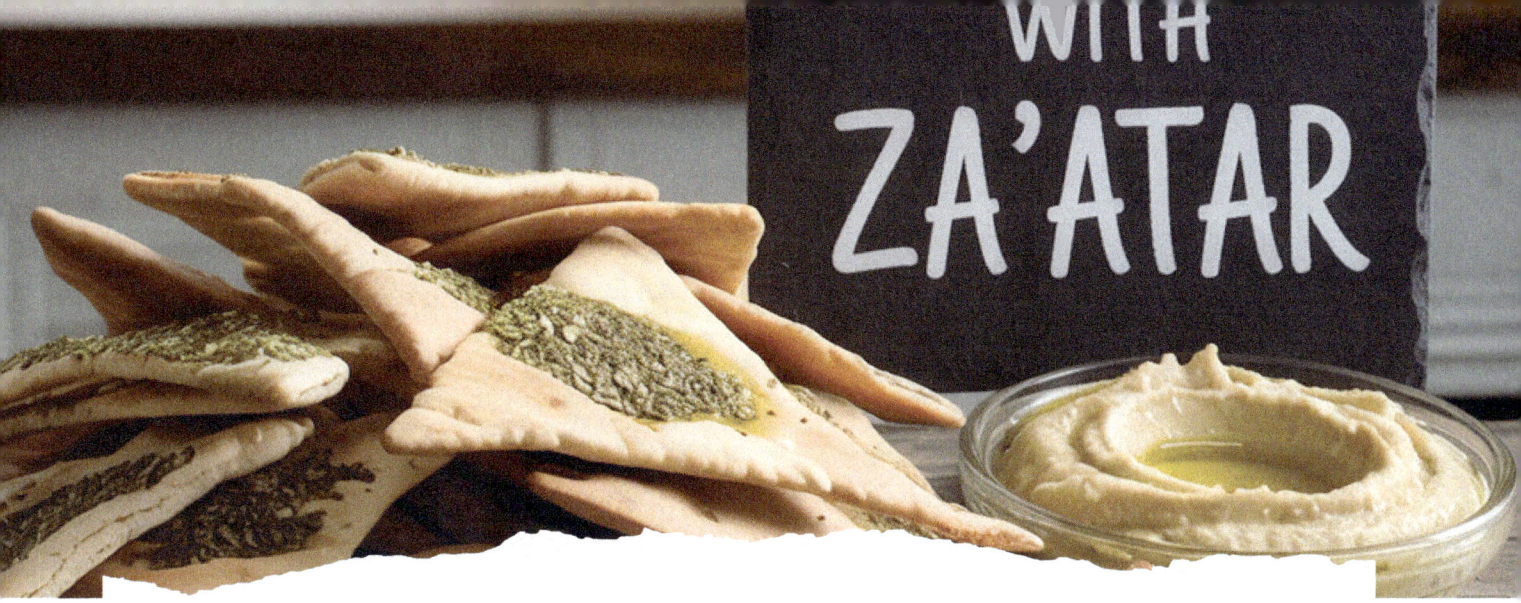

PITA CHIPS WITH ZA'ATAR

Servings: 4 **Total Time:** 15 Min

Calories: 180 | **Fat:** 9g | **Carbohydrates:** 22g | **Protein:** 4g

Ingredients

- 4 whole wheat pita breads
- 3 tablespoons extra-virgin olive oil
- 1½ tablespoons za'atar spice blend
- ½ teaspoon sea salt

Directions

- Pair these chips with hummus, baba ganoush, or tzatziki for a satisfying Mediterranean snack.
- Store leftover chips in an airtight container at room temperature for up to 3 days.
- For extra crunch, leave the chips in the oven (turned off) for 5 minutes after baking.

Tips

- Pair these chips with hummus, baba ganoush, or tzatziki for a satisfying Mediterranean snack.
- Store leftover chips in an airtight container at room temperature for up to 3 days.
- For extra crunch, leave the chips in the oven (turned off) for 5 minutes after baking.

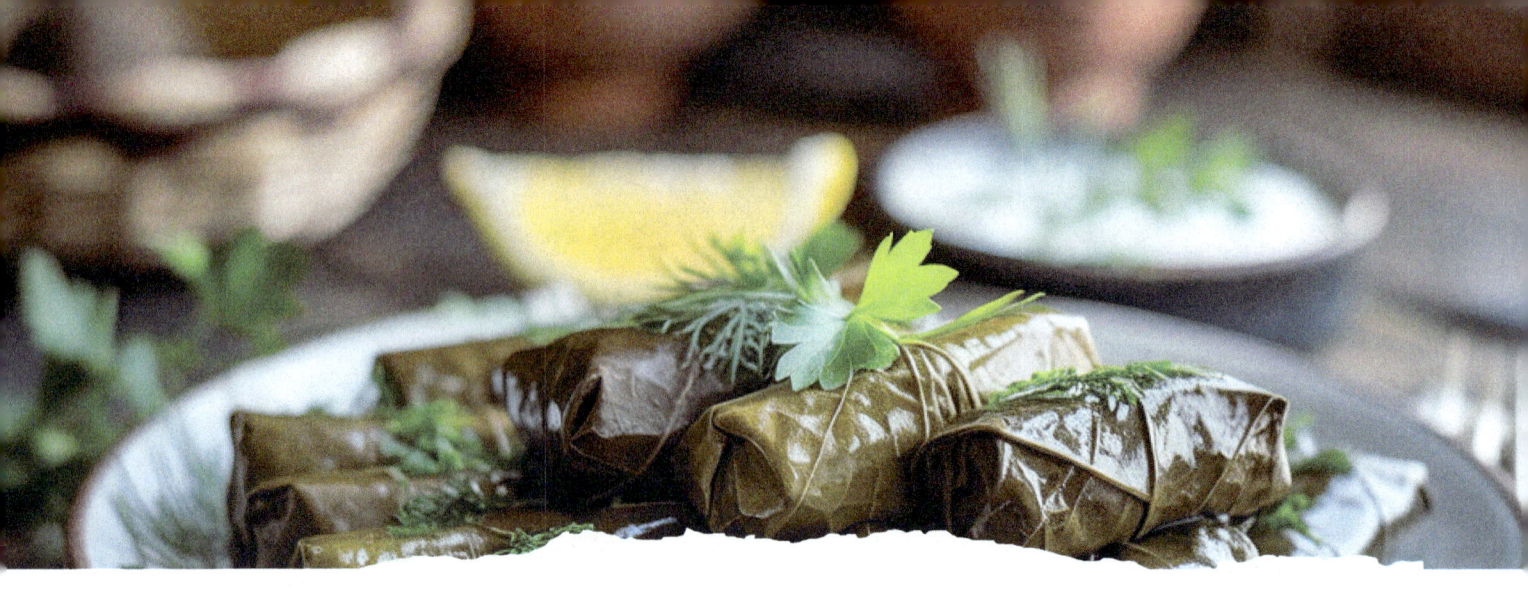

STUFFED GRAPE LEAVES (DOLMAS)

Servings: 6 | **Total Time:** 30 Min

Calories: 180 | **Protein:** 3g | **Carbohydrates:** 22g | **Fat:** 9g

Ingredients

- 1 jar (16 oz) grape leaves in brine, rinsed and drained
- 1 cup uncooked white rice (short-grain preferred)
- 1 medium onion, finely chopped
- 1/4 cup fresh parsley, chopped
- 1/4 cup fresh mint, chopped
- 1/4 cup fresh dill, chopped
- Juice of 2 lemons
- 1/3 cup olive oil (plus extra for drizzling)
- Salt and pepper to taste
- 2 cups water or vegetable broth

Tips

- You can add pine nuts or currants to the filling for added texture and sweetness.
- Use brown rice for a whole grain option (adjust cook time accordingly).
- Dolmas can be served warm or cold, and they store well in the fridge for 3–4 days.
- If grape leaves are tough, blanch them in hot water for 2–3 minutes before stuffing.

Directions

- Prepare the Filling: In a mixing bowl, combine uncooked rice, chopped onion, parsley, mint, dill, lemon juice, olive oil, salt, and pepper. Mix well.
- Stuff the Leaves: Place a grape leaf (vein side up) on a flat surface. Add about 1 teaspoon of filling near the stem end. Fold in the sides and roll up tightly, like a burrito. Repeat with remaining leaves and filling.
- Arrange and Cook: Line the bottom of a large saucepan with a few unused or torn grape leaves to prevent sticking. Arrange the stuffed leaves seam side down in layers.
- Simmer: Add water or broth to cover the dolmas. Place a heat-safe plate on top to keep them from unrolling. Cover the pot and simmer on low heat for 40–45 minutes, or until rice is fully cooked.
- Serve: Let cool to room temperature. Drizzle with olive oil and serve with lemon wedges or a side of Greek yogurt.

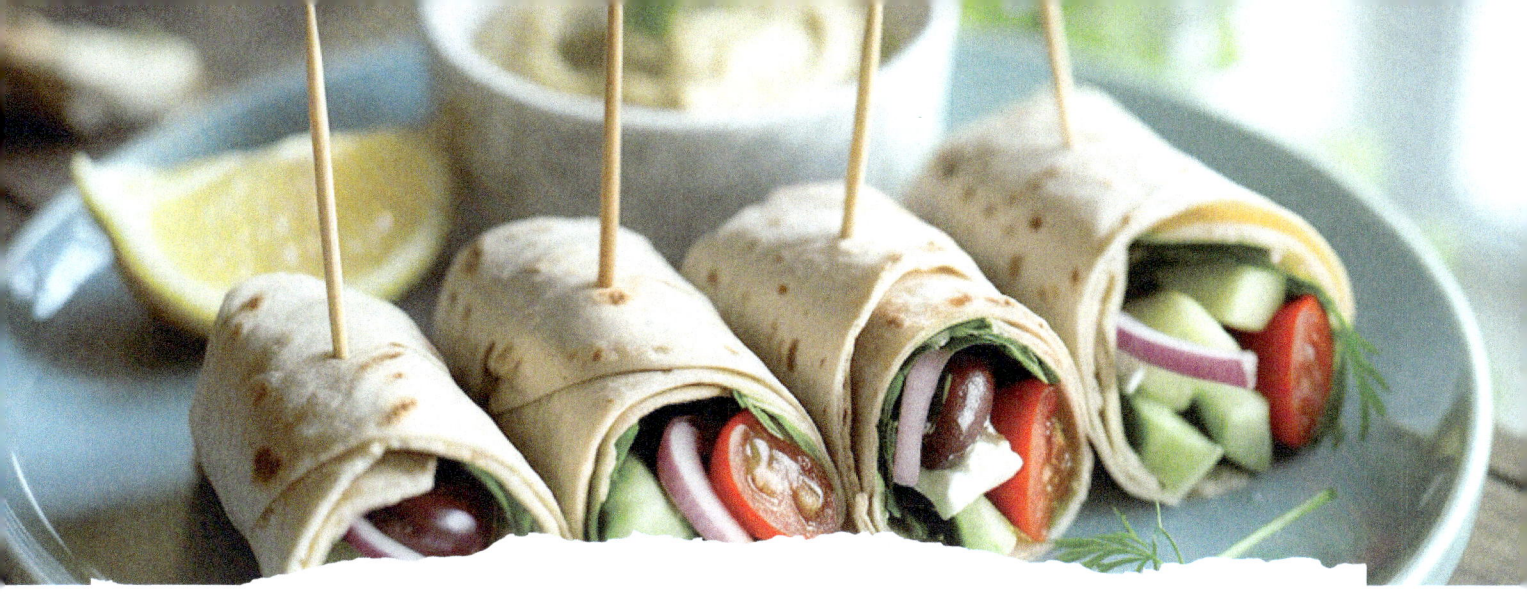

MINI GREEK VEGGIE WRAPS

Servings: 4 **Total Time:** 15 Min

Calories: 180 | **Protein:** 5g | **Carbohydrates:** 20g | **Fat:** 9g

Ingredients

- 4 small whole wheat tortillas or pita bread
- ½ cup hummus (any flavor)
- 1 cup chopped cucumber
- ½ cup cherry tomatoes, halved
- ¼ cup red onion, thinly sliced
- ¼ cup kalamata olives, pitted and sliced
- ¼ cup crumbled feta cheese
- 1 cup mixed greens or baby spinach
- 1 tbsp extra virgin olive oil
- Juice of ½ lemon
- Salt and pepper to taste

Directions

- In a small bowl, toss the chopped cucumber, tomatoes, red onion, and olives with olive oil, lemon juice, salt, and pepper.
- Lay each tortilla flat and spread a layer of hummus over the surface.
- Add a handful of mixed greens or spinach on top of the hummus.
- Spoon the veggie mixture evenly across each tortilla.
- Sprinkle with crumbled feta cheese.
- Carefully roll or fold each tortilla into a mini wrap. Secure with toothpicks if needed.
- Serve immediately or wrap in parchment for on-the-go meals.

Tips

- For extra flavor, use roasted red pepper hummus or add a dash of oregano.
- Make these ahead and store in an airtight container in the fridge for up to 24 hours.
- Want to add protein? Include grilled chicken or chickpeas.
- Perfect for seniors: soft tortillas make them easy to chew and assemble.

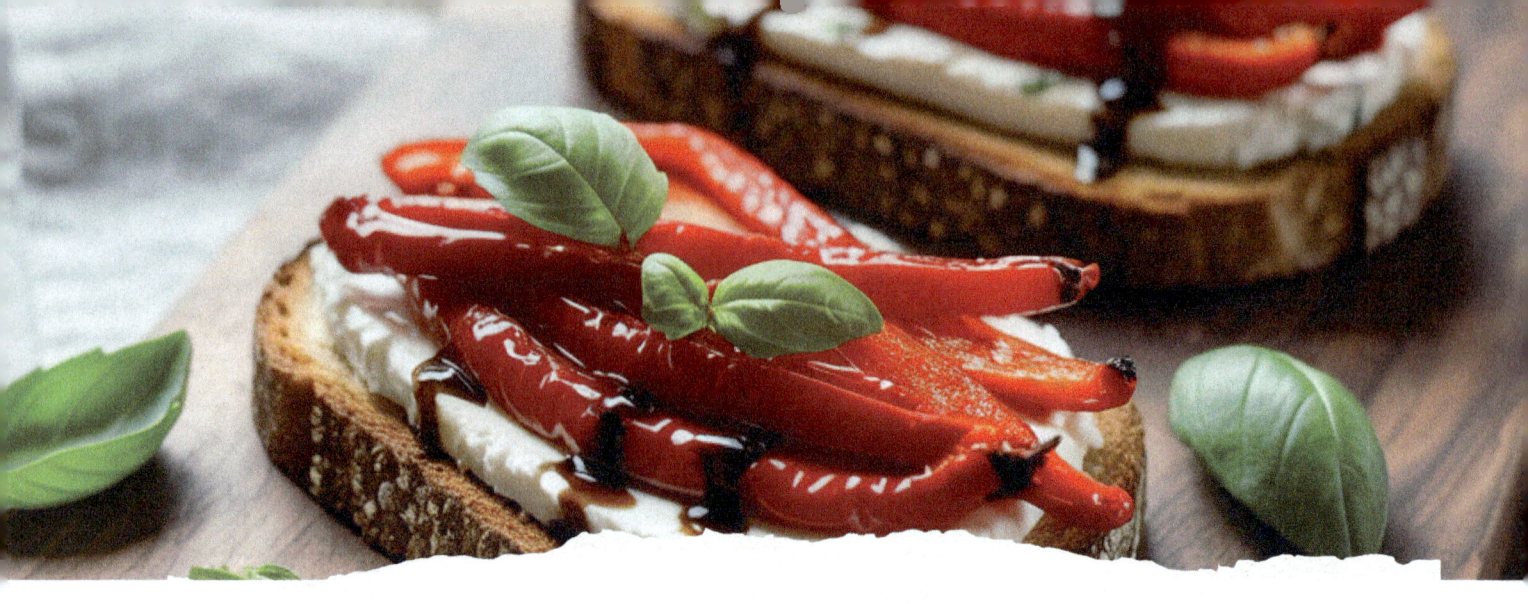

ROASTED RED PEPPER AND GOAT CHEESE TOASTS

Servings: 2   **Total Time:** 15 Min

Calories: 280 | **Protein:** 8g | **Carbohydrates:** 28g | **Fat:** 15g

Ingredients

- 4 slices of whole grain or sourdough bread
- 2 roasted red bell peppers (jarred or homemade), sliced into strips
- 4 oz goat cheese, softened
- 1 tbsp extra virgin olive oil
- 1 garlic clove, peeled
- 1 tsp balsamic glaze (optional)
- Fresh basil leaves, for garnish
- Pinch of sea salt and black pepper

Directions

- Toast the Bread: Lightly toast the bread slices in a toaster or on a skillet until golden and crisp.
- Prepare the Garlic Rub: While still warm, gently rub each slice of toast with the garlic clove for a hint of flavor.
- Spread the Goat Cheese: Evenly spread the softened goat cheese over each slice.
- Add Roasted Peppers: Top the goat cheese with slices of roasted red pepper.
- Drizzle and Season: Drizzle with olive oil (and balsamic glaze if using). Sprinkle with salt and pepper.
- Garnish: Finish with a few fresh basil leaves for a pop of color and flavor. Serve immediately.

Tips

- For homemade roasted peppers, char them over a flame or bake at 450°F until blistered, then peel.
- Swap goat cheese for feta if preferred.
- Serve as a light lunch, appetizer, or pair with a soup or salad for a complete meal.

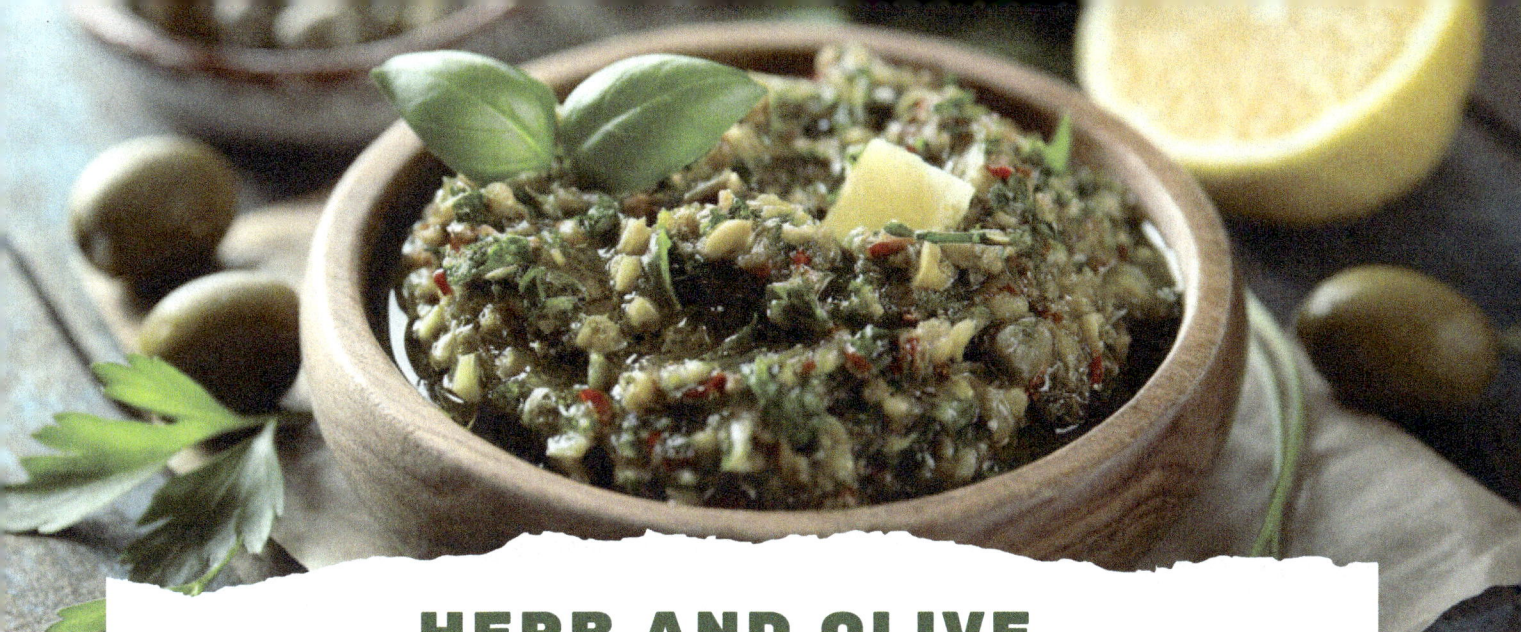

HERB AND OLIVE TAPENADE

Servings: 6   **Total Time:** 10 Min

Calories: 110 | **Fat:** 10g | **Saturated Fat:** 1.5g | **Carbohydrates:** 3g | **Protein:** 1g

Ingredients

- 1 cup mixed olives (green and black), pitted
- 2 tablespoons capers, drained
- 2 garlic cloves
- 2 tablespoons fresh parsley, chopped
- 1 tablespoon fresh basil leaves (optional)
- 1 tablespoon lemon juice
- 3 tablespoons extra virgin olive oil
- Freshly ground black pepper, to taste

Directions

- In a food processor or blender, combine the olives, capers, garlic, parsley, and basil.
- Pulse a few times until the mixture is finely chopped but still has some texture.
- Add the lemon juice and olive oil. Blend again until it reaches a spreadable consistency.
- Taste and season with black pepper if needed.
- Transfer to a bowl and serve immediately or chill for later use.

Tips

- Serve with whole-grain crackers, fresh veggies, or toasted bread.
- For a smoother tapenade, blend longer and add a little more olive oil.
- Store in an airtight container in the fridge for up to 5 days.
- Add sun-dried tomatoes or anchovies for extra flavor depth.

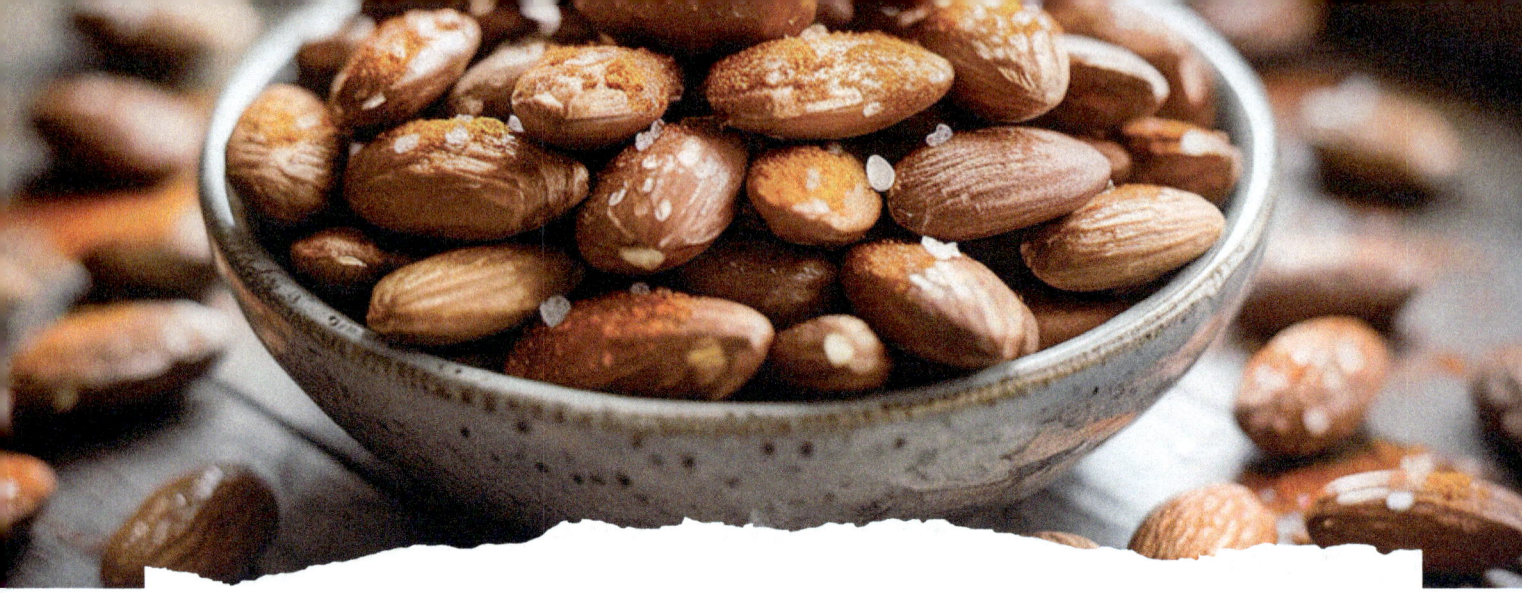

SPICED ALMONDS WITH SEA SALT

Servings: 4 | **Total Time:** 15 Min

Calories: 190 | **Protein:** 6g | **Carbohydrates:** 6g | **Fat:** 16g

Ingredients

- 1 ½ cups raw almonds
- 1 tablespoon extra-virgin olive oil
- 1 teaspoon smoked paprika
- ½ teaspoon ground cumin
- ¼ teaspoon cayenne pepper (optional for a little heat)
- ½ teaspoon garlic powder
- ½ teaspoon sea salt

Directions

- Preheat your oven to 350°F (175°C).
- In a medium bowl, combine the almonds, olive oil, paprika, cumin, cayenne (if using), and garlic powder. Toss well to coat the almonds evenly.
- Spread the almonds out on a baking sheet lined with parchment paper.
- Roast in the preheated oven for 10–12 minutes, stirring once halfway through, until the almonds are golden and fragrant.
- Remove from the oven and immediately sprinkle with sea salt while still warm.
- Allow to cool completely before serving or storing in an airtight container.

Tips

- For a sweeter version, reduce the cayenne and add a pinch of cinnamon and a drizzle of maple syrup before baking.
- These almonds make a great snack or a crunchy topping for salads and grain bowls.
- Be sure not to overbake – almonds can go from perfectly toasted to burned quickly, so keep an eye on them!

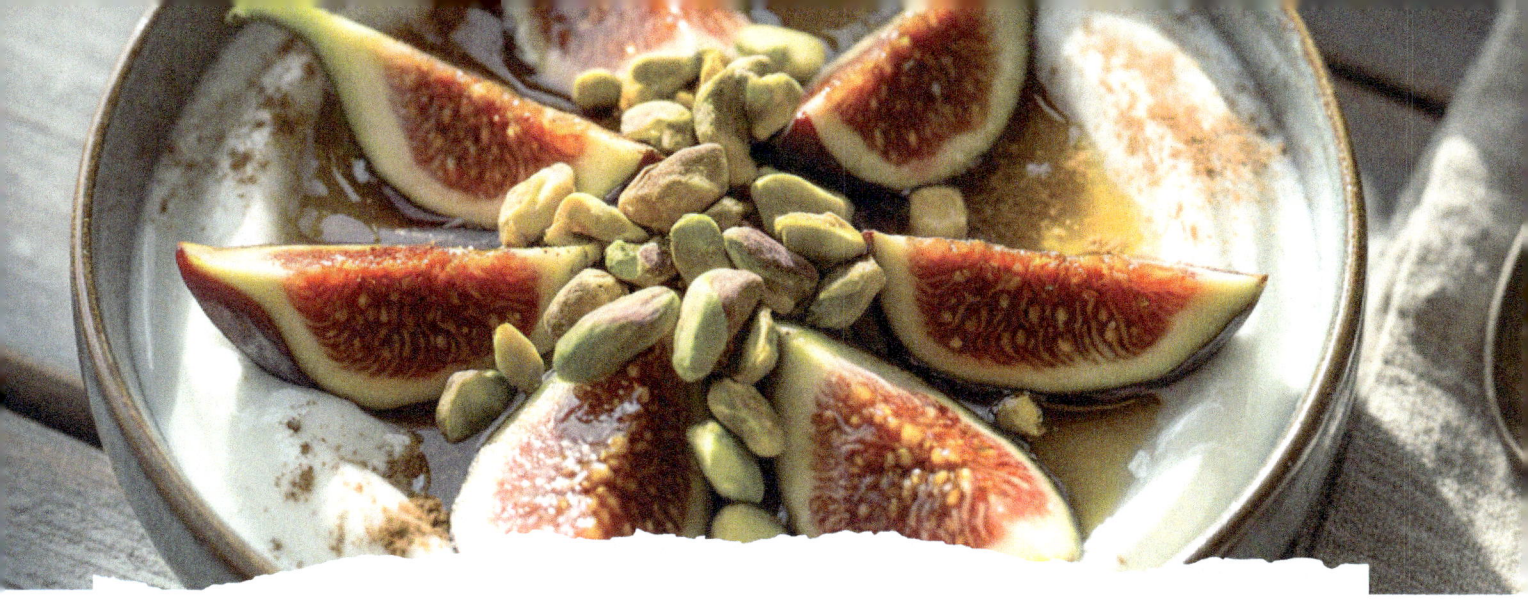

YOGURT WITH HONEY, FIGS, AND PISTACHIOS

Servings: 2 **Total Time:** 10 Min

Calories: 220 | **Protein:** 10g | **Carbohydrates:** 25g | **Fat:** 9g

Ingredients

- 1 cup plain Greek yogurt (unsweetened)
- 4 fresh figs, sliced (or 4 dried figs, chopped)
- 2 tablespoons raw honey
- 2 tablespoons chopped pistachios
- ½ teaspoon ground cinnamon

Directions

- In two small bowls or glasses, divide the Greek yogurt evenly.
- Drizzle 1 tablespoon of honey over each portion.
- Top with sliced or chopped figs.
- Sprinkle chopped pistachios over the top.
- Finish with a pinch of cinnamon if desired.
- Serve immediately and enjoy this refreshing, nutrient-rich dish.

Tips

- For extra crunch, toast the pistachios lightly in a dry pan before adding.
- Use dried figs if fresh ones aren't in season—just soak them in warm water for 10 minutes to soften.
- This makes a great healthy dessert or breakfast, and can be layered into a parfait for visual appeal.
- You can swap honey for date syrup or maple syrup for a different flavor profile.

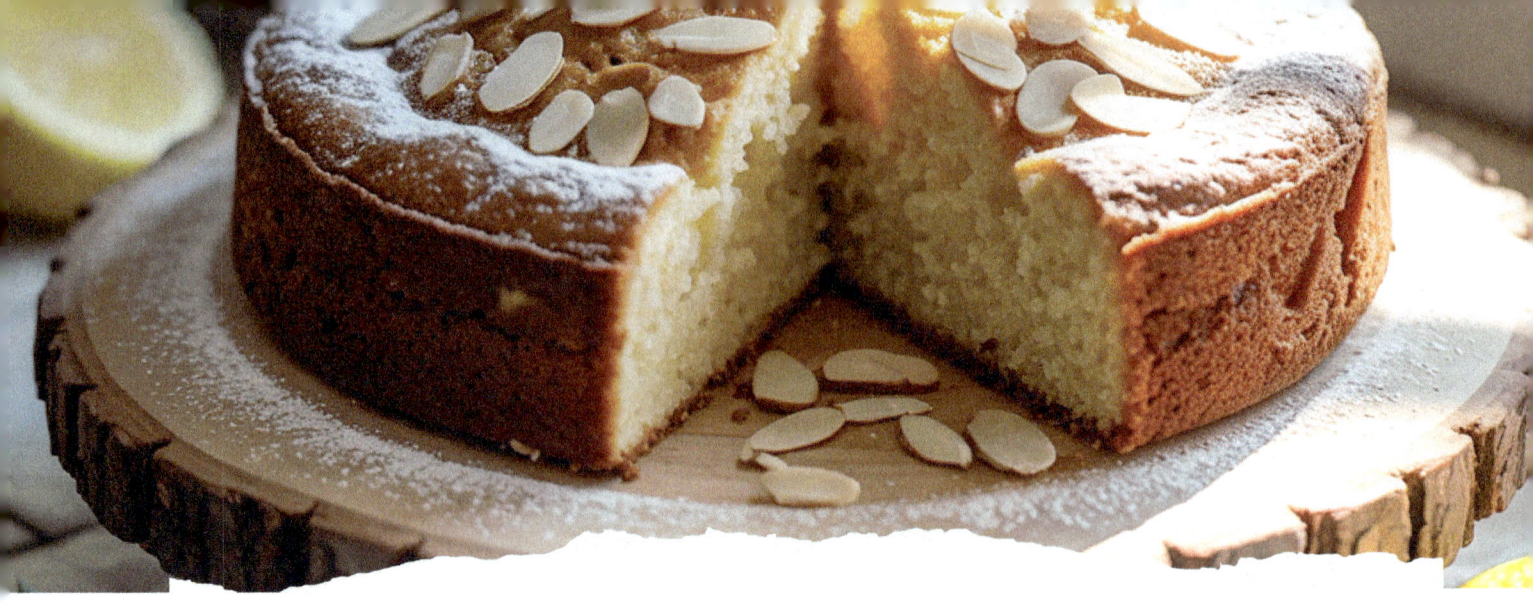

ALMOND OLIVE OIL CAKE

Servings: 8 **Total Time:** 50 Min

Calories: 280 | **Fat:** 18g | **Carbohydrates:** 25g | **Protein:** 6g

Ingredients

- 1 cup almond flour
- 1 cup all-purpose flour
- ¾ cup sugar
- ½ teaspoon baking soda
- ½ teaspoon baking powder
- ¼ teaspoon salt
- 3 large eggs
- ½ cup extra virgin olive oil
- ½ cup plain Greek yogurt
- 1 teaspoon vanilla extract
- Zest of 1 lemon
- 2 tablespoons sliced almonds

Directions

- Preheat your oven to 350°F (175°C). Grease a 9-inch round cake pan and line the bottom with parchment paper.
- In a large bowl, whisk together almond flour, all-purpose flour, sugar, baking soda, baking powder, and salt.
- In another bowl, whisk the eggs, olive oil, Greek yogurt, vanilla extract, and lemon zest until smooth.
- Pour the wet ingredients into the dry and stir until just combined – do not overmix.
- Pour the batter into the prepared pan and smooth the top. Sprinkle with sliced almonds, if using.
- Bake for 35–40 minutes, or until a toothpick inserted into the center comes out clean.
- Let the cake cool in the pan for 10 minutes, then transfer to a wire rack to cool completely.

Tips

- Use high-quality extra virgin olive oil for a richer flavor.
- This cake pairs well with fresh berries or a dollop of Greek yogurt on top.
- Can be stored in an airtight container for up to 3 days at room temperature.

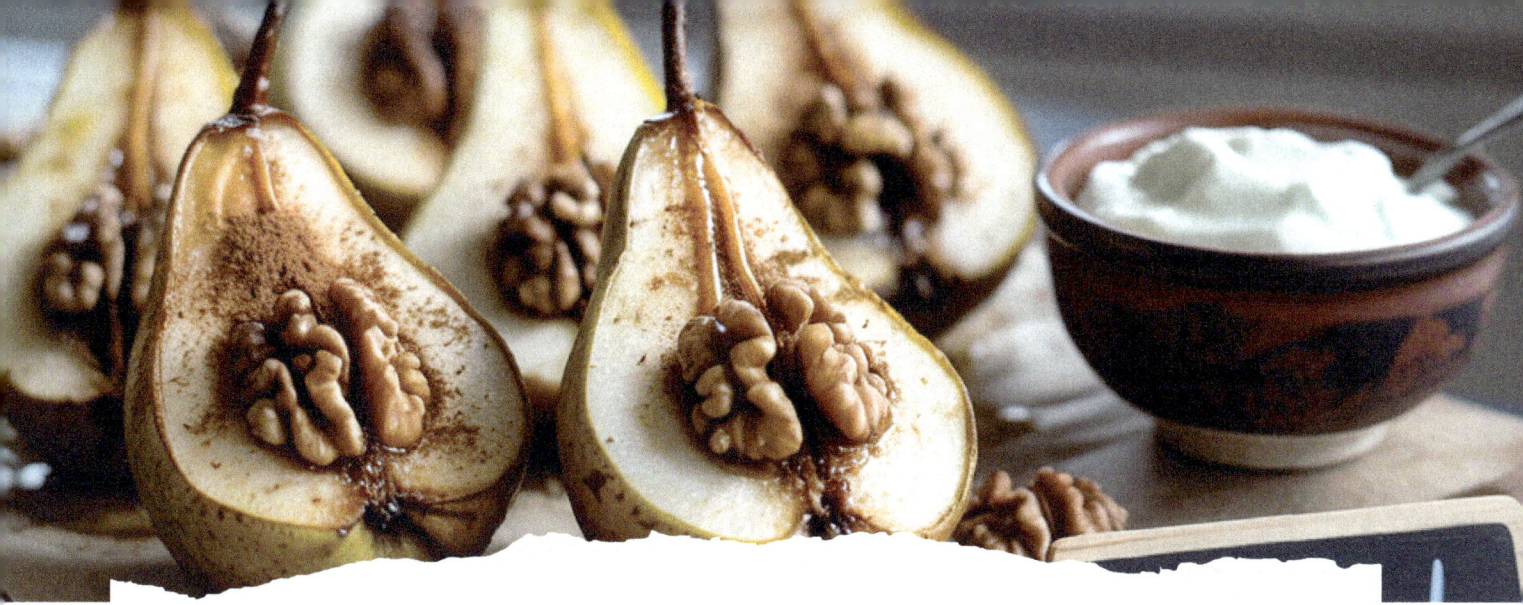

BAKED PEARS WITH WALNUTS AND CINNAMON

Servings: 2 | **Total Time:** 30 Min

Calories: 180 | **Protein:** 2g | **Carbohydrates:** 25g | **Fat:** 9g

Ingredients

- 2 ripe but firm pears, halved and cored
- ¼ cup chopped walnuts
- 1 tablespoon honey or maple syrup
- ½ teaspoon ground cinnamon
- 1 tablespoon unsalted butter (optional, for extra richness)
- A pinch of sea salt
- Plain Greek yogurt or a dollop of ricotta (optional, for serving)

Directions

- Preheat your oven to 375°F (190°C).
- Place the pear halves cut side up in a small baking dish.
- In a small bowl, mix chopped walnuts, cinnamon, and a pinch of sea salt.
- Spoon the walnut mixture into the center of each pear half.
- Drizzle the pears with honey or maple syrup. Add a small dab of butter on top of each if desired.
- Cover the baking dish with foil and bake for 20 minutes.
- Uncover and bake for an additional 5–10 minutes, or until the pears are soft and golden.
- Serve warm with a spoonful of Greek yogurt or ricotta on top (optional).

Tips

- Choose pears like Bosc or Anjou for best texture when baked.
- For a more indulgent version, add a drizzle of dark chocolate after baking.
- This makes a perfect light dessert or a naturally sweet breakfast.
- To make it vegan, use maple syrup and skip the butter or use a plant-based alternative.

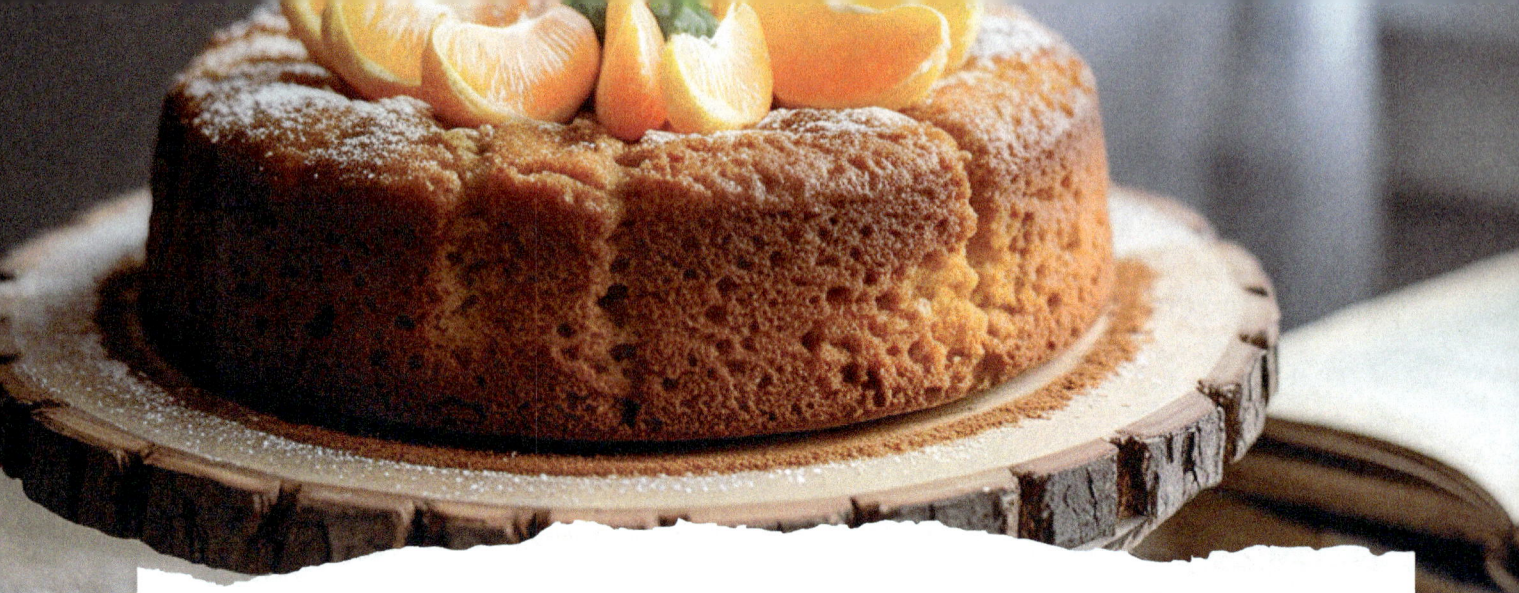

SEMOLINA ORANGE CAKE (LOW-SUGAR)

Servings: 3 | **Total Time:** 50 Min

Calories: 180 | **Protein:** 4g | **Carbohydrates:** 22g | **Fat:** 9g

Ingredients

- 1 cup semolina
- 1/2 cup plain Greek yogurt
- 1/4 cup olive oil
- 1/4 cup fresh orange juice
- 1 tablespoon orange zest
- 2 eggs
- 1/4 cup honey (or maple syrup for a vegan option)
- 1 teaspoon baking powder
- 1/2 teaspoon baking soda
- 1/2 teaspoon vanilla extract
- A pinch of salt

Directions

- Preheat the oven to 350°F (175°C). Lightly grease a 9-inch round cake pan.
- In a mixing bowl, whisk together the yogurt, olive oil, orange juice, honey, eggs, orange zest, and vanilla extract until smooth.
- In a separate bowl, combine the semolina, baking powder, baking soda, and salt.
- Slowly add the dry ingredients to the wet ingredients, stirring until just combined.
- Pour the batter into the prepared cake pan and smooth the top with a spatula.
- Bake for 30–35 minutes or until a toothpick inserted in the center comes out clean.
- Let cool completely before slicing. Serve plain or with a dusting of powdered cinnamon if desired.

Tips

- For extra moisture, brush the cake with a little warm orange juice after baking.
- This cake stores well in the refrigerator for up to 4 days.
- To make it gluten-free, use a certified gluten-free semolina or swap with almond flour (texture will vary).

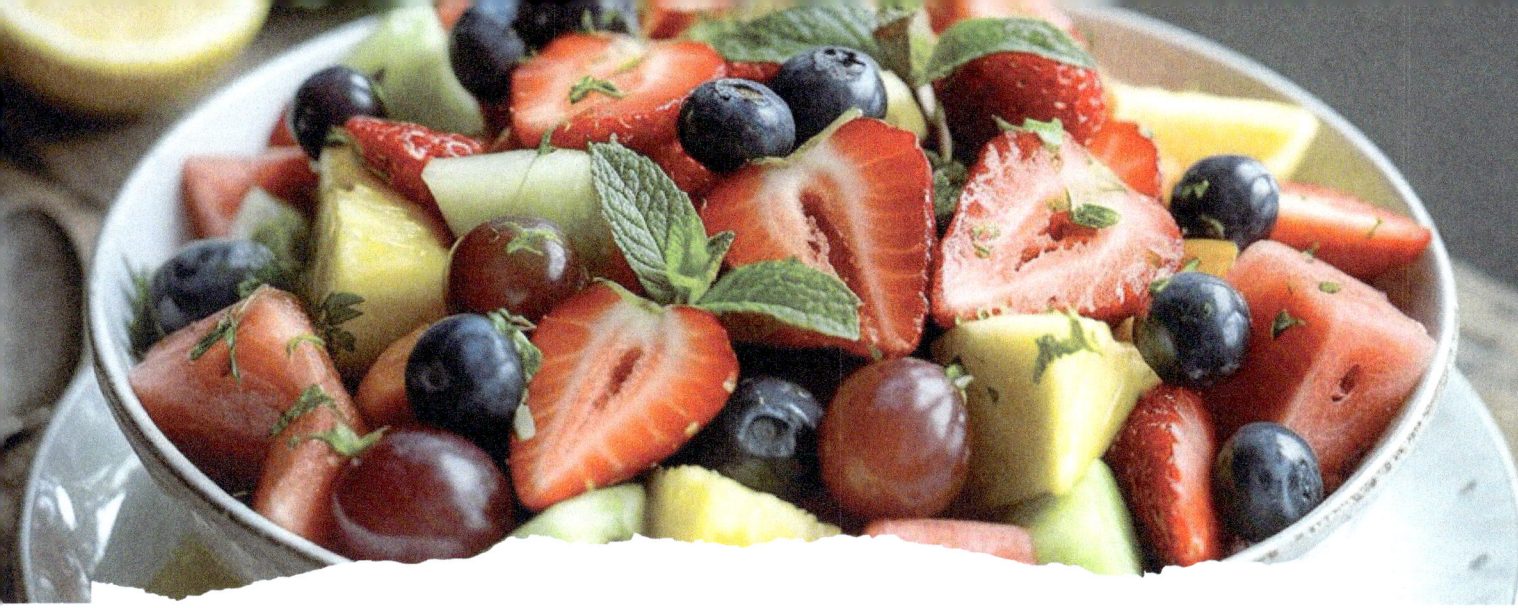

FRESH FRUIT SALAD WITH MINT AND LEMON

Servings: 4 | **Total Time:** 15 Min

Calories: 110 | **Carbohydrates:** 27g | **Protein:** 1g | **Fat:** 0.5g

Ingredients

- 1 cup strawberries, hulled and sliced
- 1 cup blueberries
- 1 cup pineapple chunks
- 1 cup watermelon, cubed
- 1 cup grapes, halved
- 1 tablespoon fresh mint leaves, finely chopped
- 1 tablespoon honey (optional)
- Juice of 1 lemon

Directions

- In a large mixing bowl, combine all the prepared fruits.
- Sprinkle the chopped mint over the fruits.
- In a small bowl, whisk together the lemon juice and honey (if using).
- Drizzle the lemon mixture over the fruit salad.
- Gently toss everything together until evenly coated.
- Chill for 10 minutes before serving, or serve immediately for a fresh treat.

Tips

- Use whatever fruits are in season or available – mango, kiwi, and oranges work great too.
- For extra crunch, sprinkle some slivered almonds or sunflower seeds before serving.
- This salad is best served fresh but can be stored in the fridge for up to 24 hours.

WEEKLY MEAL PLAN

Week 1

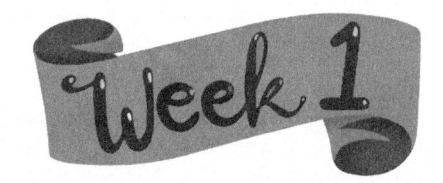

	BREAKFAST	LUNCH	DINNER	SNACK
MON	Couscous with Dried Fruits	Bulgur Wheat with Herbs and Feta	Falafel with Yogurt Sauce	Marinated Olives with Lemon and Garlic
TUE	Tomato & Spinach Egg Muffins	Eggplant Parmesan (Baked, Not Fried)	Shrimp Skewers with Garlic and Paprika	Roasted Red Pepper & Goat Cheese Toast
WED	Overnight Oats with Figs and Almonds	Falafel wrap with tahini sauce	Orzo with Roasted Peppers and	Garlic Roasted Cauliflower
THU	Greek Yogurt with Honey and Walnuts	Tuna and white bean salad	Eggplant and zucchini pasta	Baked Pears with Walnuts & Cinnamon
FRI	Olive Oil Banana Bread	Lemon Garlic Chicken Stew	Lemon herb baked cod with couscous	Fresh Fruit Salad with Mint
SAT	Smoothie with Berries, Yogurt, and Chia Seeds	Chickpea and Tuna Salad	Chickpea and Olive Pasta	Spiced Almonds with Sea Salt
SUN	Greek Yogurt with Honey and Walnuts	Tomato Basil Chickpea Stew	Herbed Chicken Thighs with Couscous	Yogurt with Honey, Figs, and Pistachios

Week 2

	BREAKFAST	LUNCH	DINNER	SNACK
MON	Mediterranean Veggie Omelet	Shrimp Skewers with Garlic and Paprika	Baked Chicken with Tomatoes and Capers	Baked Feta and Olives
TUE	Scrambled Eggs with Fresh Herbs	Grilled Lemon Herb Salmon	Lemon Garlic Chicken Stew	Roasted chickpeas
WED	Tomato & Spinach Egg Muffins	Barley Risotto with Mushrooms	Rosemary Garlic Turkey Cutlets	SPICED ALMONDS
THU	Overnight Oats with Figs and Almonds	Salmon with Cucumber-Dill Sauce	Ratatouille with lentils	Pita Chips with Za'atar
FRI	Avocado Toast with Feta and Tomatoes	Mediterranean tuna wrap	Chickpea and Sweet Potato Curry	Herb and Olive Tapenade
SAT	Breakfast Couscous with Dried Fruits	Mediterranean Tuna Patties	Chicken and Eggplant Bake	Fruit Salad with Mint and Lemon
SUN	Mediterranean Veggie Omelet	Chickpea & Olive Pasta	Stuffed zucchini boats	Almond Olive Oil Cake

Week 3

	BREAKFAST	LUNCH	DINNER	SNACK
MON	Whole Grain Pita with Hummus and Cucumbers	Cauliflower and Chickpea Soup	Ground Turkey and Veggie Skillet	Spiced Almonds with Sea Salt
TUE	Overnight Oats with Figs and Almonds	Mediterranean Fish Stew	Lemon Oregano Grilled Chicken	Almond Olive Oil Cake
WED	Couscous with Dried Fruits	Anchovy and Roasted Pepper Flatbread	Baked Chicken with Tomatoes and Capers	Stuffed Grape Leaves
THU	Smoothie w/Berries, Yogurt & Chia Seeds	Caprese salad with crusty bread	Mediterranean Chicken and Lentils	Marinated Olives
FRI	Greek Yogurt with Honey and Walnuts	Baked Feta with Cherry Tomatoes	Quinoa and Roasted Vegetable Salad	Spiced Almonds
SAT	Tomato & Spinach Egg Muffins	Grilled Chicken with Tzatziki	Hearty Lentil and Spinach Soup	Fresh Fruit Salad with Mint
SUN	Olive Oil Banana Bread	Lentil and sweet potato stew	Chickpea and Olive Pasta	Spiced Roasted Chickpeas

Week 4

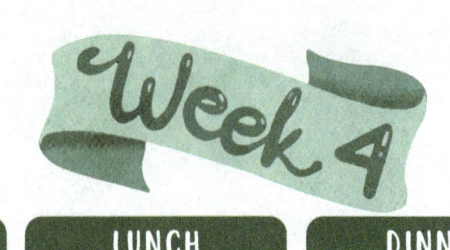

	BREAKFAST	LUNCH	DINNER	SNACK
MON	Breakfast Couscous with Dried Fruits	Chickpea shawarma bowl	Stuffed peppers with bulgur	Baked Pears with Walnuts Cinnamon
TUE	Mediterranean Veggie Omelet	Spinach and chickpea stew	Baked Cod with Tomatoes and Olives	Fruit Salad with Mint
WED	Smoothie with Berries, Yogurt, and Chia Seeds	Lentil Salad with Feta and Herbs	Shrimp and zucchini skewers	Semolina Orange Cake
THU	Scrambled Eggs with Fresh Herbs	Falafel and couscous salad	Tuna and tomato pasta	Spiced Almonds
FRI	Greek Yogurt with Honey and Walnuts	Tuna and White Bean Skillet	Eggplant and Zucchini Stew	Yogurt with Honey, Figs, and Pistachios
SAT	Avocado Toast with Feta and Tomatoes	Caprese Salad with Balsamic Glaze	Grilled Lemon Herb Salmon	Spiced Roasted Chickpeas
SUN	Olive Oil Banana Bread	Orzo with Roasted Peppers and Spinach	Chickpea and Sweet Potato Curry	Baked Feta and Olives

CONCLUSION

As we conclude our journey through the Mediterranean lifestyle tailored for seniors, it's clear that embracing this way of living offers more than just dietary changes—it fosters a holistic approach to well-being. By incorporating fresh, wholesome foods and mindful eating habits, seniors can experience enhanced vitality, improved heart health, and a greater sense of community.

Transitioning to this lifestyle doesn't require drastic changes. Small, consistent steps—like choosing olive oil over butter, savoring meals with loved ones, and incorporating more fruits and vegetables—can lead to significant health benefits. Remember, it's not about perfection but about making choices that support your health and happiness.

We at LifeQuest Publishing are honored to have been part of your journey toward a healthier, more vibrant life. Embrace the Mediterranean way, and may it bring you joy, health, and a renewed zest for life.

Enjoyed **Mediterranean Meals Made Easy for Seniors**? ✸

Would you be willing to help someone else discover it, too?

If this book has been helpful or inspiring, please consider leaving a quick review—or even just a ★★★★★ rating.

Your feedback truly makes a significant difference.

To share your thoughts, scan the code below.

-
Thank you so much for your sup

Printed in Dunstable, United Kingdom